MCQs for ENT

D1586960

MCQs for ENT
Preparation for the FRCS (ORL-HNS)

Second Edition

Edited by

Stuart Winter MD, MB, ChB, BSc, FRCS (ORL-HNS)
Consultant Ear, Nose, and Throat Surgeon, Honorary Senior Clinical Lecturer, Oxford, UK

Declan Costello MA, MBBS, FRCS (ORL-HNS)
Consultant Ear, Nose, and Throat Surgeon, Wexham Park Hospital, UK

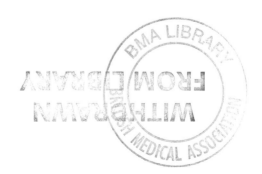

OXFORD
UNIVERSITY PRESS

OXFORD
UNIVERSITY PRESS

Great Clarendon Street, Oxford, OX2 6DP,
United Kingdom

Oxford University Press is a department of the University of Oxford.
It furthers the University's objective of excellence in research, scholarship,
and education by publishing worldwide. Oxford is a registered trade mark of
Oxford University Press in the UK and in certain other countries

© Oxford University Press 2019

The moral rights of the authors have been asserted

First Edition Published in 2008
Second Edition published in 2019

Impression: 1

Published in the United States of America by Oxford University Press
198 Madison Avenue, New York, NY 10016, United States of America

British Library Cataloguing in Publication Data

Data available

Library of Congress Control Number: 2019937236

ISBN 978–0–19–879200–0

Printed in Great Britain by
Ashford Colour Press Ltd, Gosport, Hampshire

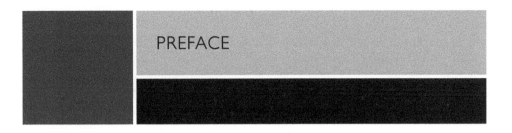

PREFACE

This book is intended as a revision aid for candidates preparing for the multiple choice question (MCQ) papers of the FRCS (ORL-HNS) examination. The style and format of the questions in the book mirrors the format of the examination questions, and covers all of the relevant topics.

The book is divided into two main sections: Single Best Answers and Extended Matching Questions.

Answers and explanatory notes are provided, along with links to relevant websites and key journal articles. In common with the examination, the book features illustrations and diagrams.

CONTENTS

List of Abbreviations   ix
Contributors   xi

Section 1: Single Best Answers

1. General Otolaryngology
Questions   3
Answers   16

2. Otology and Neuro-otology
Questions   25
Answers   38

3. Head and Neck Surgery
Questions   47
Answers   73

4. Paediatric Otolaryngology
Questions   87
Answers   100

5. Rhinology
Questions   107
Answers   125

Section 2: Extended Matching Questions

6. General Otolaryngology
Questions   141
Answers   150

7. Otology and Neuro-otology
Questions   157
Answers   164

8. Head and Neck Surgery
Questions   171
Answers   179

9. Paediatric Otolaryngology
Questions   185
Answers   192

10. Rhinology
Questions   197
Answers   205

Index   211

ABBREVIATIONS

CO_2	carbon dioxide
ENT	ear, nose, and throat
ABR	auditory brainstem response
ACE	angiotensin-converting enzyme
ADC	apparent diffusion coefficient
AHI	apnoea–hypopnea index
AJCC	American Joint Committee on Cancer
BAHA	bone-anchored hearing aid
BCC	basal cell carcinoma
BMI	body mass index
BPPV	benign paroxysmal positional vertigo
cANCA	cytoplasmic antineutrophil cytoplasmic antibody
CER	cortical evoked response
CNS	central nervous system
CRS	chronic rhinosinusitis
CSF	cerebrospinal fluid
CT	computed tomography
DVLA	Driver and Vehicle Licensing Agency
DWI	diffusion-weighed imaging
ECG	electrocardiogram
ECoG	electrocochleography
FNA	fine needle aspiration
FNAC	fine needle aspiration cytology
FRCS	Fellowship of the Royal Colleges of Surgeons
GnRH	gonadotropin-releasing hormone
GP	general practitioner
GPA	granulomatosis with polyangiitis
HPV	human papillomavirus
IAM	internal auditory meatus
IJV	internal jugular vein
KTP	potassium titanyl phosphate

MDT	multidisciplinary team
MEN	multiple endocrine neoplasia
MLB	microlaryngoscopy and bronchoscopy
MRI	magnetic resonance imaging
MTC	medullary thyroid carcinoma
NF	neurofibromatosis
NHSP	newborn hearing screening programme
NICE	National Institute for Health and Care Excellence
NICU	neonatal intensive care unit
OAE	otoacoustic emission
OPG	orthopantomogram
ROL-HNS	otorhinolaryngology-head and neck surgery
OSA	obstructive sleep apnoea
pANCA	perinuclear antineutrophil cytoplasmic antibody
PET	positron emission tomography
RCT	randomized controlled trial
RDI	respiratory distress index
SCC	squamous cell carcinoma
SDH	succinate dehydrogenase
SNHL	sensorineural hearing loss
TSH	thyroid-stimulating hormone
UK	United Kingdom
US	ultrasound *or* United States
UV	ultraviolet
VEMP	vestibular evoked myogenic potential

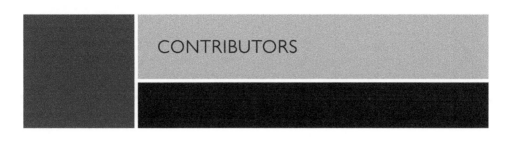

CONTRIBUTORS

Authors

Rhinology

Mr Andrew T. Harris *PhD, FRCS (ORL-HNS), Consultant Otorhinolaryngologist—Head and Neck Surgeon, Bradford Teaching Hospitals NHS Foundation Trust*

Mr S. Mark Taylor *MD, FRCS(C), FACS, Professor and Head, Otolaryngology-Head and Neck Surgery, Dalhousie University, Halifax, Canada*

Head and Neck

Mrs Lisa Fraser *FRCS (ORL-HNS), Consultant ENT Surgeon, Oxford, UK*

Paediatrics

Ms Sonia Kumar *FRCS (ORL-HNS), Consultant ENT Surgeon, Oxford, UK*

Otology and NeuroOtology

Mr Charlie Huins *MSc, FRCS (ORL-HNS), Consultant ENT and Cochlear Implant Surgeon, Queen Elizabeth Hospital, Birmingham, UK*

Additional contributions:

Mr Charles Daultrey *FRCS (ORL-HNS), Consultant ENT and Head and Neck Surgeon, Worcester, UK*

Ms Laura Jackson *PhD, FRCS (ORL-HNS), Consultant ENT Surgeon, Wolverhampton, UK*

Mr Alistair Mitchell-Innes *BSc, FRCS (ORL-HNS), International Otology Fellow, Royal Victorian Eye & Ear Hospital, Melbourne, Australia*

Section 1

SINGLE BEST ANSWERS

1. **Stimulation of which of the following nerves does not cause referred otalgia?**
   A. Glossopharyngeal nerve
   B. Descendens hypoglossi nerve
   C. Vagus nerve
   D. Lingual nerve
   E. Buccal nerve

2. **Parasympathetic innervation to the submandibular gland is carried by the:**
   A. Lesser petrosal nerve
   B. Facial nerve
   C. Glossopharyngeal nerve
   D. Jacobsen's nerve
   E. Greater superficial petrosal nerve

3. **Which of the following statements best describes the physiological regulation of saliva?**
   A. Basal saliva production is predominantly from the parotid gland
   B. Parasympathetic stimulation decreases salivary flow
   C. The parotid gland contains largely mucinous cells
   D. Saliva is produced in two stages and its ionic content is modified by the intercalated duct cells
   E. Anticholinergic drugs increase the production of saliva

4. **Which of the following statements best describes the physiology of olfaction?**
   A. The primary neuron cell body for the first cranial nerve is located in the olfactory bulb
   B. Noxious stimuli from the posterior nasal cavity are detected by the glossopharyngeal nerve
   C. The vomeronasal organ detects tactile sensation from passing odorants
   D. Each olfactory receptor expresses only one G protein receptor
   E. Olfactory receptor neurons do not regenerate

5. **What is the single most common cause of an incorrect blood transfusion being administered?**
   A. Laboratory error
   B. Error in blood donor centre
   C. Minor antigen reaction
   D. Clerical error by doctor
   E. Failure in pre-transfusion bedside checking

6. **Concerning the development of the ossicular chain, which statement best describes the first branchial arch derivatives?**
   A. The stapes develops from the first branchial arch
   B. The malleus and incus develop from the first branchial arch
   C. The head and neck of the malleus, and the body and short process of the incus develop from the first branchial arch
   D. The manubrium of the malleus and the long process of the incus develop from the first branchial arch
   E. The head of the malleus and the long process of the incus develop from the first branchial arch

7. **Concerning the pharmacokinetics of local anaesthetics, which of the following statements is false?**
   A. Lidocaine acts to reversibly block sodium channels in the nerve fibre
   B. Lidocaine acts to cause vasoconstriction when injected subcutaneously
   C. Alcoholic cirrhosis can reduce the metabolism of bupivacaine
   D. Local anaesthetics with a low pKa have a faster onset of action
   E. 8.4% sodium bicarbonate added to 2% cocaine speeds up the onset of action

8. **Which nerves pass through the superior orbital fissure?**
   A. II, III, IV, and VI
   B. III, IV, V2, and VI
   C. III, IV, V1, and VI
   D. II, IV, V2, and VI
   E. III, IV, V1, and V2

9. **Which of the following muscles do not have an attachment to the mastoid process?**
   A. Digastric
   B. Splenius capitis
   C. Longissimus capitis
   D. Temporalis
   E. Anterior auricular

10. Concerning lasers in ENT, which if any of the following statements is false?

A. The 'E' in the LASER acronym stands for 'emission'

B. The carbon dioxide (CO_2) laser emits light in the far infrared spectrum and has a wave length of 10,600 nm

C. The light generated by a laser is characterized by being monochromatic, collimated, and coherent

D. The effects of the argon laser are due to heat generated locally

E. The potassium titanyl phosphate (KTP) laser can be used in middle ear surgery and directed into small recesses by bending the laser light with a prism

11. Concerning the hyoid bone, which of the following statements is false?

A. The lesser cornu of the hyoid is derived from the second branchial arch

B. The hyoid bone is incompletely ossified at birth

C. The hyoglossus and middle constrictor muscles attach to the greater cornu

D. The intermediate tendon of the digastric muscle passes between the bifurcated tendon of the stylohyoid

E. The geniohyoid muscle acts to depress the larynx during swallowing

12. Concerning immunoglobulins, which of the following statements is false?

A. IgG crosses the placenta

B. IgG forms the largest subclass of immunoglobulins

C. Immunoglobulins are composed of heavy and light chains

D. IgA is secreted into the saliva

E. The antibody binding site is found on the heavy chain

13. Which of the following statements is true?

A. *Clostridium* are Gram-negative anaerobes

B. Some species of *Clostridium* produce an exotoxin that inhibits the sympathetic nervous system

C. *Staphylococcus aureus* are Gram-positive cocci that are arranged in clusters

D. Lancefield group C streptococci include *Streptococcus pyogenes*

E. *Treponema pallidum* is a Gram-positive spirochaete bacterium

14. In designing a trial comparing primary surgery against primary chemoradiotherapy for head and neck cancer, which of the following statements concerning randomization is true?

A. The number of patients in each arm will be the same

B. The clinician can favour one treatment over another if the patient expresses choice

C. The clinician will not be aware of which treatment the patient has received

D. The patients in each arm should have similar prognostic factors

E. Randomization ensures that there is no bias between the groups

15. A new screening test for a squamous cell carcinoma is developed. In total, 150 people were tested. Within the whole study, 50 patients were known to have the disease. When testing was started, 40 patients who tested positive had the disease, while ten patients who tested positive did not have the disease. Which of the following statements is correct?

A. The specificity of the test is 80%
B. The sensitivity of the test is 80%
C. The positive predictive value of the test is 90%
D. The negative predictive value of the test is 80%
E. The prevalence of squamous cell carcinoma in this study is 40%

16. Concerning the p-value, which of the following statements is true?

A. A p-value of 0.001 with a significance level set at 0.05 indicates that the null hypothesis is wrong
B. For a p-value to be significant it must be a value less than 0.05
C. A type I error is to reject the null hypothesis when it is true
D. A p-value of 0.0001 indicates a highly significant clinical finding
E. The null hypothesis should be rejected if the p-value is 0.1 when the significance level has been set at less than 0.05

17. Concerning statistical testing, which of the following statements is false?

A. Parametric tests make an assumption about the population distribution
B. Standard error of a population is calculated as the standard deviation divided by the square root of the population size
C. Specificity relates to the number of true positives in a test
D. A type 1 error is to reject the null hypothesis when it is true
E. A type 2 error is to accept the null hypothesis when it is false

18. A 73-year-old woman with a history of metastatic hypopharyngeal squamous cell carcinoma presents with lethargy, vomiting, hypotension, and tachycardia. A corrected serum calcium is found to be 3.14 mmol/L (2.12–2.62). Which of the following electrocardiogram (ECG) abnormalities is most likely to be found?

A. QRS interval shortening
B. QT interval prolongation
C. QT interval shortening
D. Peaked T waves
E. Poor R-wave progression

19. Which of the following statements concerning botulinum toxin is false?

A. It is produced by *Clostridium botulinum*, a Gram-positive anaerobe

B. Botulinum toxin acts at presynaptic cholinergic neuromuscular end plates by inhibiting the release of acetylcholine

C. Strains of *Clostridium botulinum* produce different antigenic toxins

D. Recovery after administration occurs as the botulinum toxin is degraded by the anticholinesterase enzyme

E. Following repeated administration, antibodies may develop that bind to the botulinum toxin inactivating it

20. Trousseau and Chvostek signs are observed in hypocalcaemia and also:

A. Hypokalaemia

B. Hyperkalaemia

C. Hypomagnesaemia

D. Hypermagnesaemia

E. Low zinc levels

21. Concerning anticancer clinical drug trials, which of the following statements is correct?

A. Phase 1 clinical trials usually involve large numbers of patients to test for anticancer properties

B. Phase 2 trials will aim to ascertain the response of the cancer to the treatment

C. A Phase 3 trial testing a new cancer drug will assess its cost-effectiveness

D. All cancer patients should be included in clinical trials

E. Patient consent is not required for the inclusion of patients with advanced cancer into phase 1 trials only

22. Which of the following statements concerning DNA (deoxyribonucleic acid) is false?

A. The base cytosine binds with guanine in DNA

B. Large parts of the human DNA sequence do not code for proteins

C. In DNA replication, DNA polymerase copies the DNA sequence in a 5′ to 3′ direction

D. Each gene's DNA sequence codes for one protein

E. RNA interference is a naturally occurring system that selectively silences individual genes

23. The optic canal is formed by which bones?

A. Frontal bone

B. Greater wing of the sphenoid

C. Lesser wing of the sphenoid

D. Temporal bone

E. Ethmoid bone

24. Parathyroid hormone has all of the following effects except:

A. Increases osteoclastic activity

B. Increases absorption of calcium from the gastrointestinal tract

C. Increases renal excretion of phosphate

D. Increases renal absorption of calcium

E. Reduces 1,25-hydroxyvitamin D3

25. In the Gell and Coombs classification, how is allergic rhinitis classified?

A. Type 1—immediate

B. Type 2—antibody dependent

C. Type 3—immune complex

D. Type 4—cell mediated

E. Type 5—seasonal

26. You are asked by the haematologists to perform a local anaesthetic biopsy of a cervical lymph node. The patient, a 45-year-old woman, has had a suspected relapse of her non-Hodgkin's lymphoma. Following her recent treatment, she is known to be thrombocytopenic. What is the LOWEST platelet count (in platelets × 10^9/L) that you would consider it acceptable to proceed with the operation?

A. 20

B. 50

C. 100

D. 150

E. 300

27. Which of the following statements can be considered false with regard to the prion protein and diseases caused by it?

A. The prion protein is expressed normally in the human brain

B. Prion diseases can be inherited, occur sporadically, or be infectious

C. An example of a human prion disease is Gerstmann–Sträussler–Scheinker disease

D. There is currently no effective treatment for prion diseases

E. In the UK, several thousand deaths have been caused by new variant Creutzfeldt–Jakob disease (nvCJD) in the last decade

28. A patient with HIV is placed on the waiting list for a parotidectomy. You are keen to warn the operating department staff of his infection risk. When the operating list is printed, which of the following is generally acceptable to use to highlight his status?

A. HIV positive

B. High-risk

C. AIDS

D. Special

E. None of the above—it is not ethical to highlight his status on a circulated list

29. **Which answer best describes the content of the cavernous sinus?**
    A. Internal carotid artery, oculomotor, trochlear, abducent, and ophthalmic and maxillary divisions of the trigeminal nerve
    B. Internal carotid artery, oculomotor, trochlear, abducent, and ophthalmic and mandibular divisions of the trigeminal nerve
    C. Internal carotid artery, superior ophthalmic vein, optic, abducent, and ophthalmic and maxillary divisions of the trigeminal nerve
    D. Common carotid artery, oculomotor, trochlear, abducent, and ophthalmic and maxillary divisions of the trigeminal nerve
    E. Superior ophthalmic vein, oculomotor, trochlear, abducent, and ophthalmic and maxillary divisions of the trigeminal nerve

30. **In the UK, in 2017 under the current Department of Health rules, when a patient is referred with suspected cancer, what is the maximum number of days (from the date of referral by the general practitioner (GP)) that a patient may wait for their definitive treatment?**
    A. 14 days
    B. 28 days
    C. 31 days
    D. 42 days
    E. 62 days

31. **Which of the following is not a recognized side effect of carbimazole?**
    A. Agranulocytosis
    B. Jaundice
    C. Alteration in sense of smell
    D. Rash
    E. Gastrointestinal symptoms

32. **The junior doctor on your team receives a complaint alleging that he was rude to a patient's daughter. What is the correct course of action?**
    A. The doctor should write a polite letter of apology
    B. You, as the doctor's senior and supervisor, should write an apology on his behalf
    C. Pass the letter to the lead clinician in your department
    D. Pass the letter to the hospital's complaints department
    E. Ask the nursing staff for a written statement about your conduct

33. **Which of the following elements of blood clotting are inhibited by the administration of warfarin?**
    A. Factors II, VII, IX, and X
    B. Factors IIa, IXa, Xa, and XIa
    C. Platelet aggregation
    D. Von Willebrand factor
    E. Factors II, VIII, and X

34. If a mother and a father are both carriers of an autosomal recessive gene, which of the following statements is true?

A. All of their children will have the disease

B. Half of their children will have the disease

C. One-quarter of the children will have the disease

D. All the males will have the disease

E. None of the children will have the disease

35. A 44-year-old man presents with a depressed left nasal bone following an alleged assault. He is noted to have reduced sensation to the nasal tip. Which nerve is likely to have been affected?

A. External nasal branch of the anterior ethmoidal nerve

B. Supratrochlear branch of the ophthalmic nerve

C. Infratrochlear branch of the ophthalmic nerve

D. Superior labial branch of the facial nerve

E. Infraorbital nerve

36. Which intrinsic laryngeal muscle is responsible for vocal cord opening?

A. Cricothyroid muscle

B. Posterior cricoarytenoid muscle

C. Lateral cricoarytenoid muscle

D. Thyroarytenoid muscle

E. Thyrohyoid muscle

37. A patient is taking warfarin for paroxysmal atrial fibrillation (PAF). Under what circumstances would it be reasonable to stop the warfarin and administer fresh frozen plasma (FFP) (or factor concentrate) and vitamin K?

A. Epistaxis controlled with anterior nasal packing

B. Epistaxis controlled only with posterior and anterior nasal packing

C. Elective admission for endoscopic sinus surgery

D. Pharyngoscopy for globus pharyngeus symptoms

E. Excision of a lipoma

38. A randomized controlled trial is conducted to evaluate a novel therapy. What level of evidence does this represent?

A. 1a

B. 1b

C. 2a

D. 2b

E. 3

39. **The CO$_2$ laser is in which class?**
    A. Class 1
    B. Class 1M
    C. Class 3B
    D. Class 4
    E. Class 2

40. **New oral anticoagulants are increasingly used for treatment and thromboprophylaxis prevention. Rivaroxaban inhibits which of the following?**
    A. Factor II
    B. Factor X
    C. Factor Xa
    D. Factor XI
    E. Factor Xia

41. **A sickle cell crisis may be precipitated by which of the following conditions?**
    A. Hypovolaemia
    B. Hypothermia
    C. Hypoxia
    D. Acidosis
    E. All of the above

42. **In regard to *Clostridium* species, which of the following statements is false?**
    A. *Clostridium tetani* produces a spastic paralysis
    B. *Clostridium botulinum* produces a spastic paralysis
    C. *Clostridium botulinum* is an obligate anaerobe
    D. In spasmodic dysphonia, type A toxin is injected into thyroarytenoid muscle
    E. *Clostridium botulinum* acts on the presynaptic nerve terminals preventing acetylcholine release

43. **Regarding the cell cycle, which of the following statements is true?**
    A. The cell cycle has five stages—G1, S, G2, M, and G0
    B. Alkylating agents work in all phases of the cell cycle by directly damaging DNA
    C. Antimetabolites work by interfering with DNA and RNA synthesis during the S phase
    D. Topoisomerase inhibitors are active through the S phase
    E. Mitotic inhibitors such as plant alkaloids prevent the S phase

44. **Regarding surgical homeostasis, which of the following statements regarding surgical homeostasis is false?**

    A. Monopolar electrocautery, the circuit is from the generator, to the active electrode through the target tissue back to the return pad which is placed on the patients
    B. Monopolar diathermy is unable to be used if a patient has a cochlear implant
    C. There are two electrodes in bipolar diathermy which forms a circuit with the return pad on the patients
    D. The harmonic scalp cuts and coagulates through high-frequency vibrations at 55,000 Hz
    E Coblation is the process whereby bipolar energy and saline form stable plasma around the electrode

45. **Which of the following statement concerning thyroid hormone synthesis is false?**

    A. Thyroid peroxidase is produced within the thyroid gland and acts to oxidize iodine and facilitate the attachment of iodine to active tyrosine units in thyroglobulin
    B. Pendrin is a potassium–chloride symporter present in the follicular cells of the thyroid gland
    C. Thyroid-stimulating hormone (TSH) is produced by the anterior pituitary gland in response to thyroid-releasing hormone from the hypothalamus
    D. TSH causes reabsorption of thyroglobulin from the follicular space
    E. Thyroid hormones triiodothyronine (T3) and thyroxine (T4) are essential for normal development

46. **Silver nitrate cautery: which of the following statements is false?**

    A. Medical silver nitrate sticks are usually purchased in combination with potassium nitrate
    B. When the applicator is combined with water, nitric acid and potassium hydroxide are produced
    C. The silver hydroxide is insoluble and produces the brownish discolouration seen with nasal cautery
    D. Any spillage on to the upper lip/facial skin should be cleaned immediately with water
    E. Uses for silver nitrate cautery include nasal cautery for epistaxis and to remove granulations around tracheal stomas

47. **Mechanism of action of antibiotics: which of these statement regarding antibiotics is false?**

    A. Human cells do not have cell walls while bacterial cells contain cell walls hence can be targeted by certain antibiotics
    B. Quinolones interfere with cell wall synthesis
    C. Sulfonamides disrupt folic acid synthesis which is an important step in the process of DNA synthesis
    D. Clavulanic acid is a beta-lactamase inhibitor which may cause a rash when administered to patients with infectious mononucleosis
    E. Vancomycin inhibits cell wall synthesis

48. **Sutures: the following statement is false?**

A. Vicryl is absorbed via hydrolysis in 55–70 days
B. The difference between Vicryl and Vicryl Rapide lies in its tensile strength which for Vicryl Rapide is 50% at 5 days
C. Silk sutures are absorbed within 2–3 months
D. Monocryl is an absorbable monofilament
E. Polypropylene has a high tensile strength and is biologically inert, therefore causing minimal tissue reaction

49. **Which of the following is least likely to be an extrapulmonary manifestation of sarcoidosis?**

A. Yellow/brown submucosal nasal nodules
B. Lupus pernio
C. Oral and palatal ulceration
D. Vertigo
E. Xerophthalmia

50. **In regard to the mechanism of swallowing, which of the following statements is false?**

A. The pharyngeal stage is the quickest and involves soft palate elevation
B. The muscles of the soft palate are all innervated by the pharyngeal plexus
C. There are three stages of swallowing: oral, pharyngeal, and oesophageal
D. The upper oesophageal sphincter is composed of striated muscle which includes cricopharyngeus and thyropharyngeus
E. The oral stage of swallowing is under voluntary control

51. **Which of the following is not a pure sensory branch of the mandibular nerve?**

A. Meningeal nerve
B. Buccal nerve
C. Auriculotemporal nerve
D. Lingual nerve
E. Inferior alveolar nerve

52. **Prior to mastoid surgery in a 100 kg man, you decide to infiltrate the postauricular area with Lignospan via a dental syringe. Each vial of Lignospan contain is 2.2 mL and contains 2% lidocaine with 1:80,000 adrenaline. How many vials can you safely use?**

A. 3
B. 5
C. 7
D. 9
E. 11

53. Which of the following signs is least likely to occur in a base of skull fracture?

A. Periorbital ecchymosis

B. Purulent otorrhoea

C. Mastoid ecchymosis

D. Watery rhinorrhoea

E. Subconjunctival haemorrhages

54. To establish whether cholesteatoma in adults is associated with smoking, which would be the most appropriate study design?

A. Randomized control trial

B. Systematic review

C. Prospective cohort study

D. Case-controlled study

E. Case report

55. Blood supply to the tonsil: which of the following arteries does not directly supply the tonsil?

A. Maxillary artery

B. Dorsal lingual arteries

C. Tonsillar artery

D. Ascending palatine artery

E. Descending palatine artery

56. Disorders of the oesophagus: which of the following statements best describes pathology affecting the oesophagus?

A. Achalasia is a primary oesophageal dysmotility disorder characterized by impaired relaxation of the upper oesophageal sphincter

B. The Z line marks the transition between stratified squamous epithelium of the oesophagus and non-secretory pseudostratified mucosa of the stomach

C. Achalasia is associated with an increase in ganglion cells of the myenteric plexus

D. Oesophageal dysmotility may present in patients with Raynaud's phenomenon and sclerodactyly

E. Gaviscon Advance contains sodium alginate and sodium bicarbonate

57. Which of the following best describes the American Society of Anesthesiologists (ASA) grade of a 72-year-old patient undergoing a mastoid exploration? He has poorly controlled diabetes with hypertension and a body mass index (BMI) of 43.

A. ASA I

B. ASA II

C. ASA III

D. ASA IV

E. ASA V

58. Which segments of the internal carotid artery do not have branches (more than one answer)?

A. Cervical segment

B. Petrous (horizontal) segment

C. Lacerum segment

D. Cavernous segment

E. Clinoid segment

1. B. The descendens hypoglossi nerve (C1) is a motor nerve. It joins the descendens cervicalis to form the ansa cervicalis, which supplies the strap muscles.

The glossopharyngeal nerve receives sensation from the posterior one-third of the tongue, the tonsils, the pharynx, and the middle ear.

The vagus nerve supplies sensation to the pinna, tympanic membrane, larynx, hypopharynx, vallecula, and the subglottis.

The lingual nerve, a branch of the mandibular division of the trigeminal nerve, supplies sensation from the anterior two-thirds of the tongue. It also carries 'hitch-hiking' taste and parasympathetic fibres from the chorda tympani.

The buccal nerve is also a branch of the mandibular division of the trigeminal nerve, and transmits sensory information from the skin over the buccal membrane and from the second and third molar teeth.

2. B. The parasympathetic supply of the submandibular gland is carried by the facial nerve. The chorda tympani branch of the facial nerve exits the skull base via the petrotympanic fissure to enter the infratemporal fossa. It then hitchhikes on the lingual nerve (branch of V3) to supply taste to the anterior two-thirds of the tongue and provide parasympathetic fibres to the submandibular gland.

The lesser petrosal nerve (continuation of Jacobsen's nerve) is a branch of the glossopharyngeal nerve. It supplies parasympathetic fibres to the parotid gland.

The greater superficial petrosal nerve branches off the facial nerve at the geniculate ganglion and is then joined by the deep petrosal nerve (sympathetic fibres). It passes forward in the pterygoid canal (Vidian canal) to give parasympathetic innervation to the lacrimal, nasal, palatine, and pharyngeal glands.

3. D. Saliva is produced in two stages. Initially it is isotonic; however, the ductal cells modify the ionic composition such that the saliva that is secreted has a similar composition to intracellular fluid.

The basal saliva production is predominantly from the submandibular gland (60–70%) with lesser contributions from the parotid (20–30%) and sublingual glands (5–10%).

When stimulated, the parotid contributes the majority of saliva production and this is predominantly regulated by parasympathetic stimulation. Therefore anticholinergic drugs reduce saliva production.

The parotid gland largely contains serous cells while the submandibular and sublingual glands contain serous and mucinous cells.

4. D. Each olfactory receptor cell expresses only one type of olfactory receptor. However, a given olfactory receptor can bind to a variety of odour molecules with varying affinities.

The primary neuron cell body for the first cranial nerve is located in the nasal mucosa. The cell is bipolar, with a dendrite extending to the nasal mucosa. The cell projects unmyelinated axons from the olfactory receptor cells towards the ipsilateral olfactory bulb to make contact with the second-order neurons.

The trigeminal nerve innervates the posterior nasal cavity to detect noxious stimuli.

The vomeronasal organ is a specialized structure located in the base of the anterior nasal septum. It is believed to have a role in detecting pheromones.

Olfactory receptor neurons are replaced approximately every 40 days.

5. E. Contrary to popular opinion, it is clinical ward mistakes that account for most erroneous blood transfusions.

6. C. The first arch derivatives of the ossicular chain are the malleus (head and neck) and the incus (body and short process). The stapes superstructure, manubrium of the malleus, and long process of the incus are derived from the second branchial arch.

7. B. Lidocaine acts to cause vasodilatation in common with other local anaesthetics except cocaine, which is a vasoconstrictor.

Local anaesthetics block sodium channels preventing depolarization and the propagation of action potentials.

Amides, including bupivacaine, are principally metabolized in the liver, therefore cirrhosis can affect its metabolism.

The speed of onset of the local anaesthetic is proportional to the concentration of non-ionized molecules. The lower the pKa, the higher the concentration of non-ionized molecules at a given pH and therefore the faster the onset of action. Sodium bicarbonate raises the pH and the speed of action.

8. C. The following structures pass through the superior orbital fissure: the lacrimal nerve (V1), frontal nerve (V1), trochlear nerve (IV), superior ophthalmic vein, nasociliary nerve (V1), inferior ophthalmic vein, abducens nerve (VI), oculomotor nerve superior division (III), and oculomotor nerve inferior division (III).

9. D. The muscles attached to the mastoid process are the digastric (posterior belly), sternocleidomastoid, splenius capitis, longissimus capitis, and the anterior, superior, and posterior auricular muscles.

The temporalis is not attached to the mastoid process.

10. E. LASER is an acronym standing for Light Amplification by the Stimulated Emission of Radiation. The light generated is characterized by being all the same colour (monochromatic), parallel (collimated), and in phase (coherent). The effects of all lasers are due to locally generated heat. The KTP laser does have a role in middle ear surgery but is delivered via total internal reflection along an optical fibre and not bent by a prism. The wavelength of the CO_2 laser is 10,600 nm.

11. E. It is the infrahyoid muscles which act to depress the larynx during swallowing.

The hyoid develops from the second and third brachial arches. The lesser cornu form the second arch and the greater cornu form the third.

Ossification begins in the body and greater cornus and is complete in adolescence.

The hyoglossus and middle constrictor attach to the greater cornu.

The digastric muscle does pass through the tendon of the stylohyoid.

12. E. The antibody binding site is part of the light chain. IgG is the only immunoglobulin to cross the placenta and makes up the largest subclass of immunoglobulins. These are composed of heavy and light chains. IgA is present in the secretions of the respiratory tract, lacrimal glands, and salivary glands.

13. C. *Clostridium* are Gram-positive anaerobes. *Clostridium botulinum* produces an exotoxin that inhibits acetylcholine release from parasympathetic muscle nerve endings. *Streptococcus pyogenes* is classified as Lancefield group A. Group C contains no significant organisms. *Treponema pallidum* is a Gram-negative spirochaete bacterium that causes syphilis.

14. D. The main purpose of randomization is that each group will have similar prognostic factors. Randomization would need to be restricted to ensure equal numbers in each group. The clinician cannot exert bias over the selection group. Comparing surgery with chemoradiotherapy, it will be obvious following treatment which arm the patient was randomized to unless the data are analysed by a blinded researcher. Randomization does not ensure that there is no bias between groups.

15. B. The following figure needs to be constructed to answer this question (bold figures are those given in the text).

		Positive	Negative	TOTAL
SCREENING	Positive	40	10	50
TEST	Negative	10	90	100
	TOTAL	**50**	100	**150**

The specificity of the test is calculated as the number of true negative results divided by the total number of patients without the disease: 90/100 (90%).

The sensitivity of the test is calculated as the number of true positive results divided by the total number of patients with the disease: 40/50 (80%).

The positive predictive value of the test is calculated as the number of true positive results divided by the total number of positive tests: 40/50 (80%).

The negative predictive value of the test is calculated as the number of true negative results divided by the total number of negative tests: 90/100 (90%).

Prevalence is calculated as the number with the disease over the sample size: 50/150 (33%).

16. C. A type 1 error is to reject the null hypothesis when it is true; this often occurs due to a small sample size.

A p-value less than the significant level set indicates that in the test the null hypothesis should be rejected. This is not the same as saying the null hypothesis is wrong. The p-value can be set at any level between 0 and 1 and is only arbitrarily set as less than 0.05 in most studies.

The null hypothesis is rejected if the p-value is smaller than or equal to the significance level.

17. C. Sensitivity refers to true positive test results and specificity to true negative results. Parametric tests make an assumption about the population distribution and assume a Gaussian or normal distribution. The standard error of a population is calculated as the standard deviation divided by the square root of the population size. A type 1 error is to reject the null hypothesis when it is true and a type 2 error is not rejecting the null hypothesis when it is false.

18. C. Hypercalcaemia can result in a variety of symptoms including fatigue, depression, confusion, anorexia, nausea, vomiting, constipation, pancreatitis, and calculi. This can be remembered using the mnemonic 'bones, stones, moans, and psychic groans'. ECG abnormalities include a shortened QT interval.

19. D. Recovery occurs through proximal axonal sprouting and muscle reinnervation by formation of new neuromuscular junctions. Botulinum toxin is produced by *Clostridium botulinum*, a Gram-positive anaerobic bacterium. Botulinum toxin is broken into seven neurotoxins. The toxin acts by binding to presynaptic sites on the cholinergic nerve terminals. This decreases the release of acetylcholine, causing a neuromuscular blockade. The botulinum neurotoxin can be immunogenic and antibodies may develop that can inactivate it.

20. C. Magnesium is the fourth most common cation in the body. The clinical effects of hypomagnesaemia are neuromuscular irritability, central nervous system (CNS) hyperexcitability, and cardiac arrhythmias, including Trousseau and Chvostek signs.

21. B. A phase 1 trial is the first stage in testing a new treatment. The trials are conducted to assess the safe dose range, side effects, and effects on the cancer. Phase 1 trials usually include only a small number of study volunteers.

Phase 2 trials are usually larger than phase 1 trials. If a phase 2 trial can show that the new treatment is as good or better than an existing treatment, then a phase 3 trial can be started. A phase 3 study is a formal comparison between the treatment results with the new therapy compared with a standard treatment. This may include a comparison of survival or side effects.

Clinical trials are certainly important, but it is the patient's choice whether they wish to be included in a trial, and consent is always required.

22. D. The concept that each gene is translated by one messenger RNA into a single protein is now understood to be false. There are in fact many proteins produced from each gene sequence.

The four bases found in DNA are adenine (A), cytosine (C), guanine (G), and thymine (T). Each type of base on one strand forms a complementary base pairing with a base on the other strand. A binding to T, and C binding to G.

The human DNA sequence contains large regions of non-coding base pairs. Only about 1.5% of the human genome consists of protein-coding exons, with over 50% of human DNA consisting of non-coding repetitive sequences. The exact role of these sequences is unknown but may be involved in the regulation of gene expression.

When a cell divides, it must replicate the DNA in its genome. The two strands are separated and the enzyme DNA polymerase creates the complementary DNA sequence. This occurs in a 5′ to 3′ direction. Transcription of the genetic sequence into mRNA (messenger RNA) and subsequently into a protein is performed by the enzyme RNA polymerase.

RNA interference (RNAi) is an RNA-dependent gene silencing process that is mediated by the RNA-induced silencing complex (RISC). This is a naturally occurring event used to regulate gene expression. The RNAi pathway has been exploited in experimental biology to study the function of genes. Using this mechanism, researchers can silence the expression of a targeted gene. This has been extremely useful in understanding the physiological role of the gene product. The use of RNAi and silencing of key genes involved in tumour development are being investigated as potential clinical therapeutic options.

23. C. The optic canal is formed by the lesser wing of the sphenoid.

24. E. Parathyroid hormone (PTH) acts to increase the circulating levels of calcium. This is achieved by increasing osteoclastic activity, stimulating the kidney to reabsorb calcium and excrete phosphate. It also acts to convert 25-hydroxyvitamin D3 to the active form 1,25-di-hydroxyvitamin D3 which stimulates the absorption of calcium from the gastrointestinal tract.

25. A. Allergic rhinitis is a type 1 hypersensitivity reaction provoked by re-exposure to a specific type of antigen.

26. B. A normal platelet count is 150–400 × 10^9/L, but it is generally considered safe to perform surgery at platelet levels of greater than 50 × 10^9/L.

27. E. Deaths in the UK attributable to nvCJD total less than 200 at present.

The human prion gene encodes a protein of amino acids and is found in most tissues of the body but is expressed at highest levels in the CNS.

Prion diseases are unique in that they can be inherited, they can occur sporadically, or they can be infectious. They can affect both animals and humans. Examples include Creutzfeldt–Jakob disease (CJD) and Gerstmann–Sträussler–Scheinker (GSS) in humans, bovine spongiform encephalopathy (BSE) in cattle, and scrapie in sheep.

All prion diseases are fatal, with no effective form of treatment currently.

28. B. The theatre staff should be alerted to his high-risk status, but it is not acceptable to state the exact reason.

29. A. The content of the cavernous sinus is the internal carotid artery, oculomotor, trochlear, abducent and ophthalmic and maxillary divisions of the trigeminal nerve.

30. E. Maximum cancer waits from time of GP referral are:

- 14 days until first appointment with specialist
- 31 days from decision to treat until first definitive treatment
- 62 days until first definitive treatment.

31. B. Relatively common side effects of carbimazole include allergic-type reactions of fever, rash, urticaria, and arthralgia. Agranulocytosis is a much-feared but rare complication of carbimazole and propylthiouracil. It occurs in 0.1–0.5% of patients and occurs suddenly. Routine monitoring of full blood count is therefore of little use.

32. D. Every hospital has a complaints department, and all disputes should be referred to them. It may be necessary to provide a written statement about the incident, but this is best handled by that department.

33. A. Vitamin K, in its reduced form, is a cofactor for the enzymatic reaction in which the glutamic acid residues on the amino terminal end of coagulation factors II, VII, IX, and X are converted into gamma-carboxyglutamic acid residues.

Warfarin acts as a competitive inhibitor of the reaction in which oxidized vitamin K is turned into reduced vitamin K.

Hence, warfarin inhibits the vitamin-K dependent factors, namely II, VII, IX, and X.

Factors IIa, IXa, Xa, and XIa are inhibited by the heparin–antithrombin complex.

Von Willebrand factor is a plasma glycoprotein that acts as a bridge between platelets and damaged subendothelium at the site of vascular injury.

34. C. Half of the children will be carriers; one-quarter will be homozygous for the gene and hence will have the disease; and one-quarter will neither be carriers nor have the disease.

35. A. Sensation to the dorsum and tip of the nose is supplied by the external nasal branch of the anterior ethmoidal nerve (V2). This emerges from between the nasal bones and the upper lateral cartilages.

36. B. The posterior cricoarytenoid muscle is the only abductor of the vocal cords.

37. B. In the elective situation, the patient's anticoagulation should be discussed with his/her cardiologist. Epistaxis requiring anterior and posterior packing suggests a heavy bleed, and it would be reasonable under these circumstances to reverse the warfarin. If the bleeding is controlled with conventional anterior packing, cessation of the warfarin will suffice.

38. B. Levels of evidence for studies evaluating therapy, prevention, aetiology, or harm:
- 1a—systematic review (with homogeneity) of randomized controlled trials (RCTs).
- 1b—individual RCT (with narrow confidence interval).
- 2a—systematic review (with homogeneity) of cohort studies.
- 2b—individual cohort study (including low-quality RCT; e.g. <80% follow-up).
- 3a—systematic review (with homogeneity) of case–control studies.
- 3b—individual case–control study.
- 4—case series (and poor-quality cohort and case–control studies).
- 5—expert opinion without explicit critical appraisal, or based on physiology, bench research, or 'first principles'.

39. D. Medical lasers are class 4.

40. C. There are three new oral anticoagulants that have been licensed for use in stroke, for thromboprophylaxis for hip and knee surgery, and for non-valvular atrial fibrillation. Apixaban and rivaroxaban are both direct, orally active, highly selective activated factor X inhibitors (Xa inhibitors). Dabigatran etexilate is a prodrug that is converted *in vivo* to the direct thrombin inhibitor dabigatran. It is a potent orally active drug that inhibits free thrombin, fibrin-bound thrombin, and thrombin-induced platelet aggregation.

41. E. The goals of anaesthesia in patients with sickle cell disease are to avoid precipitants of sickle cell crisis (hypoxia, vascular stasis, hypothermia, hypovolaemia, and acidosis), optimize perioperative pain control, and monitor for a vaso-occlusive crisis, an acute chest syndrome, an aplastic crisis, and a splenic sequestration syndrome.

42. B. *Clostridium tetani* produces a spastic paralysis while *Clostridium botulinum* produces a flaccid paralysis. The botulinum toxin binds to presynaptic terminals preventing acetylcholine release at the neuromuscular junction. *Clostridium tetani* produces exotoxins which bind to peripheral nerve terminals It is then transported through retrograde axonal transport to the CNS where it binds to presynaptic inhibitory nerve endings to block the release of inhibitory neurotransmitters across the neuromuscular junction.

43. A. The cell cycle has multiple stages. During G1 the cell prepares for division. DNA synthesis occurs, replicating the genetic material in the S phase and the chromosomes now consist of two sister chromatids. During the G2 phase, the cell assembles cytoplasmic materials necessary for the M phase where nuclear division (karyokinesis/mitosis) and cell division (cytokinesis) occur. Chemotherapeutic agents work by targeting different phases of the cell cycle to alter and arrest growth of malignant cells.

44. C. Monopolar electrosurgery: the active electrode is placed in the entry site and can be used to cut tissue and coagulate bleeding. The return electrode pad is attached to the patient, so the electrical current flows from the generator to the electrode through the target tissue, to the patient return pad and back to the generator.

Bipolar electrosurgery uses lower voltages so less energy is required and the electrosurgical current in the patient is restricted to just the tissue between the arms of the forceps electrode.

45. B. Iodide in the blood is taken up by follicular cells by a sodium–iodide symporter and then transported in to the follicular space by pendrin—an iodide chloride symporter/antiporter. Here it is oxidized to iodine, attached to active tyrosine units in thyroglobulin to form thyroid hormone precursors. Under the action of TSH, thyroglobulin is reabsorbed back in to the follicular cells and iodinated tyrosines are cleaved to form thyroid hormones, mainly T4. Pendred syndrome is an autosomal recessive condition characterized by a mutation in the *PDS* gene, which codes for the pendrin symporter. As well as being expressed in the thyroid gland, pendrin is also found in the cochlea and kidney.

46. B. When the applicator is combined with water, nitric acid and silver hydroxide are produced. It is the silver hydroxide that causes the brownish discolouration seen.

47. B. Penicillin is an inhibitor of cell wall synthesis. Bacteria have peptidoglycan-based cell walls. Antibiotics that inhibit cell wall synthesis prevent peptidoglycan synthesis, rendering these cells vulnerable to osmotic lysis. Quinolones such as ciprofloxacin inhibit nucleic acid synthesis by inhibiting DNA gyrases or topoisomerases required for DNA coiling.

48. C. Silk was one of the first non-absorbable sutures used. It is a natural suture produced from silkworm and is treated with silicone for strength and to allow easy passage through tissues. The advantages of silk include being easy to handle, a good ability to hold knots, and low tissue reactivity.

49. D. Sarcoidosis is a multisystem granulomatous condition affecting the lungs and mediastinum with 30–40% of cases displaying extrapulmonary manifestations and 10–15% otolaryngological manifestations. These include cutaneous, sinonasal, laryngeal, and cervical pathology. Salivary gland pathology can range from xerostomia to facial nerve palsy and Heerfordt syndrome. Acoustic and vestibular symptoms have been reported as a result of brainstem and therefore cranial nerve infiltrations but are rare.

50. B. There are five paired muscles of the soft palate: tensor veli palatine, levator veli palatine, palatoglossus, palatopharyngeus, and the muscle of the uvula. All are innervated by the pharyngeal plexus except tensor veli palatine, which is innervated by the mandibular branch of the trigeminal nerve.

51. E. The inferior alveolar nerve is not a pure sensory nerve. It provides a motor branch to the mylohyoid muscle before entering the mandibular canal.

52. E. The safe dose of lidocaine with adrenaline is 7 mg/kg (3 mg/kg without adrenaline) to a maximum dose of 500 mg. Each vial of Lignospan contains 44 mg, therefore 11 vials can be used.

53. B. While many base of skull fractures may be asymptomatic, signs include periorbital ecchymosis (raccoon eyes), cerebrospinal fluid (CSF) rhinorrhoea, CSF otorrhoea, haemotympanum, mastoid ecchymosis (Battle's sign), and cranial nerve dysfunction. These should all be actively looked for in any patients with significant head injury and suspicion of a fracture.

54. D. A case-controlled study is useful for the study of diseases, especially rare diseases. The patients with the disease are identified and their past exposure to aetiological factors is assessed. A longitudinal study (cohort study) is used to study risk factors. These may be prospective or retrospective depending on when the disease develops compared with recruitment in to the study, that is, a prospective cohort study looks at a group of individuals who have been exposed and follows them over time to see if disease develops. In a retrospective cohort study, some of the individuals have already developed disease and the investigators go back to identify the cohort and find information about their exposure.

55. A. The arterial supply of the tonsils is derived from the descending palatine artery, the ascending pharyngeal artery, the tonsillar branch of the facial artery, the ascending palatine artery, and the dorsal lingual branch of the lingual artery. Venous blood drains through the lingual and pharyngeal veins in to the internal jugular vein.

56. D. Achalasia is a primary oesophageal dysmotility disorder characterized by impaired relaxation of the lower oesophageal sphincter. Most commonly there is a decrease in ganglion cells of the myenteric (Auerbach's) plexus. CREST syndrome is characterized by calcinosis, Raynaud's phenomenon, oesophageal dysmotility, sclerodactyly, and telangiectasia.

57. C.

Table 1.1 American Society of Anesthesiologists (ASA) grade

ASA I	**A** normal, healthy patient: healthy, non-smoking, no or minimal alcohol use
ASA II	**A** patient with mild systemic disease: mild diseases only without substantive functional limitations. Examples include (but are not limited to) current smoker, social alcohol drinker, pregnancy, obesity (30< BMI <40), well-controlled DM/HTN, mild lung disease
ASA III	**A** patient with severe systemic disease: substantive functional limitations; one or more moderate to severe diseases. Examples include (but are not limited to) poorly controlled DM or HTN, COPD, morbid obesity (BMI ≥40), active hepatitis, alcohol dependence or abuse, implanted pacemaker, ESRD undergoing regularly scheduled dialysis, premature infant PCA <60 weeks, history (>3 months) of MI, CVA, TIA, or CAD/stents
ASA IV	**A** patient with severe systemic disease that is a constant threat to life: examples include (but are not limited to) recent (<3 months) MI, CVA, TIA, or CAD/stents, ongoing cardiac ischaemia or severe valve dysfunction, sepsis, DIC
ASA V	**A** moribund patient who is not expected to survive without the operation: examples include (but are not limited to) ruptured abdominal/thoracic aneurysm, massive trauma, intracranial bleed with mass effect
ASA VI	**A** declared brain-dead patient whose organs are being removed for donor purposes

BMI, body mass index; CAD, coronary artery disease; COPD, chronic obstructive pulmonary disease; CVA, cerebral vascular accident; DIC, disseminated intravascular coagulation; DM, diabetes mellitus, ESRD, end-stage renal disease; HTN, hypertension; MI, myocardial infarction; PCA, postconceptual age; TIA, transient ischaemic attack.

Data from http://www.asahq.org.

58. A, C, E

The 1996 Bouthillier classification describes the internal carotid artery according to the seven segments visible on angiography rather than its embryology.

1. **Which of the following is not an opening into the temporal bone?**
   A. Internal auditory canal
   B. Vestibular aqueduct
   C. Jugular foramen
   D. Cochlear aqueduct
   E. Subarcuate fossa

2. **Which of the following best describes Koerner's septum?**
   A. The petrosquamous suture
   B. The squamotympanic suture
   C. The petrotympanic suture
   D. The medial limit of the mastoid antrum
   E. The bony covering of the sigmoid sinus

3. **An auditory brainstem implant is being inserted into a patient with neurofibromatosis type 2. Where is the target region for the implant?**
   A. On the floor of the third ventricle
   B. The cochlear nucleus
   C. The olivary complex
   D. The vestibular nuclei
   E. The inferior colliculus

4. **When performing a middle cranial fossa approach for an acoustic neuroma, which of the following is the least useful surgical landmark?**
   A. Middle meningeal artery
   B. Greater superficial petrosal nerve
   C. Arcuate eminence
   D. Bill's bar
   E. Foramen ovale

5. **Which answer best describes the anatomy of the vestibular system?**
   A. The superior vestibular nerve is anterior to the facial nerve in the internal auditory canal
   B. Surgical division of the superior vestibular nerve is a recognized treatment for benign paroxysmal positional vertigo (BPPV)
   C. Vestibular evoked myogenic potentials (VEMPs) exploit a vestibulocollic reflex whose afferent limb is the superior vestibular nerve
   D. The utricle principally senses linear acceleration in a horizontal plane
   E. The principal arterial supply to the vestibular organs is from the middle meningeal artery

6. **Which of the following statements best describes electrophysiological brainstem response audiometry?**
   A. The auditory brainstem response (ABR) is a measure of the cochlear response to a stimulus
   B. During ABR testing, wave one (I) represents activity in the cochlear nucleus
   C. Electrocochleography (ECoG) provides an accurate assessment of auditory thresholds at low frequencies
   D. ECoG can accurately test for Ménière's disease
   E. Cortical evoked response (CER) audiometry requires the non-test ear to be masked

7. **Cochlear anatomy and physiology: which of the following statements is false?**
   A. Endolymph has an electrolyte composition similar to intracellular fluid (high potassium and low sodium ions)
   B. There are equal numbers of outer and inner hair cells
   C. The inner hair cells receive 95% of the afferent innervation from the cochlear nerve
   D. The stereocilia act as mechanical transducers
   E. Inner hair cells are arranged in a single row

8. **A man has been sitting on a playground roundabout facing the centre of rotation and travelling in a clockwise direction. When the roundabout stops, he has fast beating nystagmus to the right. Which of the following statements is correct?**
   A. He has ampullopetal flow of endolymph in his left superior semicircular canal
   B. He has ampullopetal flow of perilymph in his left posterior semicircular canal
   C. He has ampullopetal flow of endolymph in his right horizontal semicircular canal
   D. He has ampullofugal flow of perilymph in his right horizontal semicircular canal
   E. He has ampullofugal flow of endolymph in his right horizontal semicircular canal

9. **Which of the following statements best describes otoacoustic emissions (OAEs)?**

   A. OAEs represent sound generated by the outer hair cells

   B. OAEs are usually present in children with glue ear

   C. A positive test is subjective based on the interpretation of the result

   D. In neonatal screening, the demonstration of OAEs excludes severe sensorineural hearing loss

   E. Evoked OAEs are generated by all normal cochleas

10. **A 45-year-old man undergoes speech audiometry. Which of the following statements is false?**

    A. Speech audiometry frequently uses spondees, that is, phonetically balanced words

    B. The speech recognition threshold is the quietest level that an individual can repeat half of the spondees

    C. If the patient developed glue ear, it is likely that his maximal discrimination score will remain the same

    D. Speech audiometry can always detect feigned hearing loss from true threshold change

    E. 'Roll over' of the speech audiogram is associated with retrocochlear pathology

11. **Concerning noise-induced hearing loss, which of the following statements is most appropriate?**

    A. The inner hair cells are more susceptible to damage than the outer hair cells

    B. Intermittent noise exposure is more harmful than continuous noise exposure at a similar frequency and intensity

    C. Noise-induced hearing loss occurs because a temporary threshold shift does not occur

    D. Hair cell regeneration takes up to 10 years

    E. A 10 dB increase in sound level involves a tenfold increase of the sound intensity

12. **The owner of a Birmingham car factory approaches you. His workers are exposed to a continuous constant level of noise. He wishes to know, at what level does he needs to provide ear protectors?**

    A. 75 dBA

    B. 80 dBA

    C. 85 dBA

    D. 90 dBA

    E. 95 dBA

13. **Which statement best describes the underlying genetic problem in neurofibromatosis type 2 (NF2)?**

A. It is an inherited autosomal dominant syndrome. There is overexpression of the tumour suppressor gene on chromosome 22

B. It is an inherited autosomal dominant syndrome. There is overexpression of the tumour suppressor gene on chromosome 17

C. It is an inherited autosomal recessive syndrome. There is overexpression of the tumour suppressor gene on chromosome 22

D. It is an inherited autosomal recessive syndrome. There is decreased expression of the tumour suppressor gene on chromosome 22

E. It is an inherited autosomal dominant syndrome. There is decreased expression of the tumour suppressor gene on chromosome 22

14. **A patient is on your operating list for a right stapedotomy. Which of the following would cause you most concern?**

A. Suppurative ear discharge

B. A tympanic membrane perforation

C. Cochlear otosclerosis on the CT scan

D. Previous stapes surgery

E. A dead left ear

15. **A 46-year-old man presents to the Accident and Emergency department following a head injury with a clear discharge from his right ear. Which of the following statements concerning beta-2 transferrin and cerebrospinal fluid (CSF) leaks is false?**

A. Beta-2 transferrin is unique to the CSF

B. The test requires only a small volume

C. Beta-2 transferrin can be detected even in the presence of contamination with blood

D. Beta-2 transferrin has a high sensitivity and specificity in diagnosing CSF leak

E. The test involves an electrochemical diffusion gradient

16. **In the recovery room following a modified radical mastoidectomy, the patient is found to have a facial nerve palsy. The surgeon was confident that she had not injured the nerve during the operation. What would be the most appropriate next action?**

A. Immediately re-explore the ear

B. Give steroids in recovery

C. Wait for the local anaesthetic to wear off

D. Ask a colleague to re-explore the ear immediately

E. Arrange a computed tomography (CT) scan

17. **Which nerve is least likely to be affected in a patient with a lesion involving their jugular foramen?**

    A. Vagus nerve
    B. Cervical sympathetic chain
    C. Spinal accessory nerve
    D. Glossopharyngeal nerve
    E. Hypoglossal nerve

18. **You are called to the Accident and Emergency department to see a 26-year-old woman who has taken an overdose of aspirin within the last 24 hours. She has developed tinnitus and has hearing thresholds of 50 dB bilaterally. Previously she reports normal hearing. What advice would you give her?**

    A. In the long term, her hearing is likely to remain constant with thresholds of 50 dB
    B. Her hearing is likely to get worse over the next few months
    C. Early consideration of a cochlear implant will give her the best chance of functional recovery
    D. Her hearing is likely to improve
    E. She is likely to need a bone conduction hearing aid in the long term

19. **A 22-year-old male presents with left pulsatile tinnitus. A CT scan is arranged. What is the likely diagnosis?**

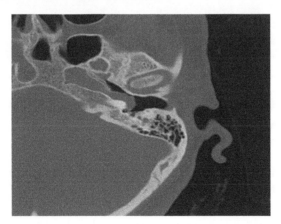

    A. Cholesteatoma
    B. Glomus tympanicum
    C. Glomus jugulare
    D. Persistent stapedial artery
    E. Carotid body tumour

20. **A 46-year-old male has a magnetic resonance imaging (MRI) scan due to asymmetrical sensorineural hearing loss and paraesthesia of his left ear canal. A high-resolution T2-weighted MRI demonstrates a large left-sided tumour in the cerebellopontine angle returning mixed signal. What is the likely cause for the altered sensation?**

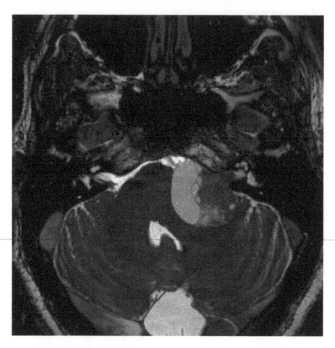

A. Compression of the superior vestibular nerve

B. Compression of the inferior vestibular nerve

C. Compression of the cochlear nerve

D. Compression of the facial nerve

E. Compression of the vagus nerve

21. **What is the most common histopathological finding associated with congenital deafness?**

A. Cochlear aplasia

B. Loss of the bony division between the apical and middle turns of the cochlea

C. Dysplasia of the membranous labyrinth

D. Partial aplasia of the cochlear duct

E. Hypoplasia of the stria vascularis

22. **Which of the following statements best describes the use of sodium fluoride in the treatment of otosclerosis?**
    A. The usual dose of sodium fluoride is 1–2 g per day
    B. Sodium fluoride has no side effects
    C. Sodium fluoride is effective at reversing established hearing loss
    D. Sodium fluoride is thought to reduce bone resorption
    E. Intratympanic sodium fluoride administration allows a more accurate dose titration

23. **The radiological imaging characteristics of a cholesterol granuloma of the temporal bone are best described as:**
    A. Hyperintense on T1 and T2 MRI
    B. Hyperintense on T1 and hypointense on T2 MRI
    C. Hypointense on T1 and hyperintense on T2 MRI
    D. Enhancement following gadolinium contrast on MRI
    E. Contrast enhancement on CT scanning

24. **Within the middle cranial fossa, the arcuate eminence on the superior aspect of the temporal bone corresponds best to which structure?**
    A. The apical turn of the cochlea
    B. The epitympanic recess of the middle ear
    C. The greater superficial petrosal nerve
    D. The superior semicircular canal
    E. The lateral aspect of the internal acoustic meatus

25. **A 46-year-old man presents with reduced hearing in his right ear. On examination he is found to have a single bony mass protruding into the ear canal with a build-up of cerumen and consequent conductive hearing loss. Clinically this is an osteoma. Which of the following statements is the least accurate description for this condition?**
    A. Osteomas are benign tumours
    B. They typically develop along the tympanosquamous or tympanomastoid suture line
    C. Surgical removal is curative
    D. Histologically, they are described as being composed of mature lamellar bone with bone marrow
    E. They are commonly associated with a history of cold water exposure

26. **Concerning the outer and middle ear sound-transformer mechanisms, which of the following statements is false?**
    A. The pinna aids in the localization of sound
    B. An in-the-ear hearing aid will generally reduce 2 kHz sounds
    C. The ratio of the size of the tympanic membrane to the stapes footplate is important in sound amplification
    D. The ossicular chain dampens sound transmission to the inner ear
    E. The middle ear transformer mechanism normally results in a 25 dB amplification of sound

27. **While descending on a SCUBA dive, a 30-year-old man experiences a sudden onset of hearing loss and vertigo. Which of the following best describes the mechanism of injury to his inner ear?**

    A. Rupture of the round window on 'Valsalva' equalization of pressure
    B. Increased middle-ear pressure on descent
    C. Ossicular discontinuity
    D. Tympanic membrane rupture
    E. Rupture of stapedius tendon

28. **A 25-year-old woman presents with a 4-day history of right-sided facial weakness. On examination, she is found to have a House–Brackmann grade IV facial palsy. No underlying cause is found, and a diagnosis of Bell's palsy is made. Regarding her recovery, what best describes her likely recovery?**

    A. There is a greater than 90% chance of a complete recovery
    B. There is approximately a 70% chance of a complete recovery
    C. There is approximately a 50% chance of a complete recovery
    D. There is approximately a 30% chance of a complete recovery
    E. There is approximately a 10% chance of a complete recovery

29. **Gentamicin is known to be ototoxic. On which part(s) of the inner ear does it exert its toxic effects?**

    A. Stria vascularis
    B. Hair cells
    C. Cochlear nerve
    D. Apical turn of cochlea
    E. Macula densa

30. **Which of the following statements regarding clival chordoma tumours is true?**

    A. The tumour arises from a remnant of the first branchial arch
    B. They occur exclusively in the head and neck
    C. Primary chemotherapy offers the best chance of survival
    D. Clival tumours are usually extradural
    E. Clival tumours commonly present with hypoglossal nerve palsy

31. **Aminoglycosides are recognized to have ototoxic properties. Which of the following statements is correct?**

    A. Aminoglycosides cause a predominantly low-frequency hearing loss
    B. Aminoglycoside toxicity usually spontaneously improves over weeks to months
    C. Mutations in the 12S mitochondrial rRNA gene are associated with low-dose aminoglycoside ototoxicity
    D. Gentamicin is more cochleotoxic than vestibulotoxic
    E. The principal area of damage is the stria vascularis

32. **Concerning barotrauma following flying, which of the following statements is false?**

    A. The Eustachian tube is normally closed
    B. Otalgia on ascent is more common than on descent
    C. The volume of air in the middle ear cleft decreases as atmospheric pressure increases
    D. Hearing loss and vertigo can occur due to the pressure changes exerted during flying
    E. Air pressure at sea level is 760 mmHg

33. **Which of the following is not an indication for placement of a bone-anchored hearing aid (BAHA)?**

    A. Congenital ossicular malformation
    B. Complete absence of the external ear (grade III microtia)
    C. Unilateral sensorineural hearing loss
    D. Bilateral sensorineural hearing loss
    E. Learning difficulties and a conductive hearing loss

34. **Which of the following statements is true of Carhart's effect?**

    A. It may occur in glue ear
    B. It typically occurs at 4 kHz
    C. It is not improved following stapes surgery
    D. It represents a genuine sensorineural hearing loss which is overcome with stapes surgery
    E. It occurs only in otosclerosis

35. **Which of the following sounds should be used when performing a visual reinforcement audiogram (VRA)?**

    A. Warble tones
    B. Pure tones
    C. White noise
    D. Complex sound (e.g. music)
    E. All of the above

36. **Which of the following best describes cholesteatoma recurrence?**

    A. A CT scan showing an epitympanic mass with a Hounsfield unit of +100
    B. A CT scan showing an epitympanic mass with a Hounsfield unit of −15
    C. A MRI scan showing an epitympanic mass that is hyperintense on diffusion-weighed imaging (DWI) with a b value of 1000 s/mm^2, and a low signal on the apparent diffusion coefficient (ADC) map
    D. A MRI scan showing an epitympanic mass that is hyperintense on DWI with a b value of 1000 s/mm^2 and a high signal on the ADC map
    E. A MRI scan showing an epitympanic mass that is hypointense on DWI with a b value of 1000 s/mm^2 and a low signal on the ADC map

37. Which of the following statements are false?

A. The *SERPINF1* gene is associated with otosclerosis
B. Tinnitus is present in around 75% of patients with otosclerosis
C. Imaging is 90% sensitive in otosclerosis
D. Mumps is a risk factor for otosclerosis
E. Otosclerotic plaques usually originate from the fissula ante fenestram

38. Which of the following is not a cause for pulsatile tinnitus?

A. Benign intracranial hypertension
B. Arteriovenous malformation
C. Glomus tympanicum
D. Patulous Eustachian tube
E. Carotid dissection.

39. Which of the following is not an indication for auditory brainstem implantation?

A. Cochlear ossification
B. Neurofibromatosis type 2
C. Michel deformity
D. Cochlear nerve aplasia
E. Mondini malformation

40. Which of the following statements is false?

A. Neurofibromatosis type 2 is associated with the merlin protein encoded by the *NF2* gene on chromosome 21
B. Vestibular schwannomas form around 80% of cerebellopontine angle tumours
C. There is a 1% risk of malignancy in vestibular schwannoma
D. The gamma knife is effective in around 95% of treated patients with vestibular schwannoma
E. Antoni type A histology shows parallel nuclei, and uniform spindle cells

41. The pars tensa develops from:

A. Ectoderm
B. Endoderm
C. Mesoderm
D. A and C
E. All three germ cell layers

42. Which of the following statements is true?

A. The pinna must be pulled posteroinferiorly to see the tympanic membrane
B. The lateral two-thirds of the external auditory canal (EAC) is cartilaginous and the medial third is cartilaginous
C. The bony labyrinth ossifies from ten centres
D. The endolymphatic sac may be found directly deep to Trautman's triangle
E. The pinna attains 90–95% of the adult size by the age of 5–6 years

43. Gradenigo syndrome is characterized by all of the following except:

A. Diplopia

B. Retro-orbital pain

C. Petrous apex abscess

D. Otorrhoea

E. Cranial nerve V and VI involvement

44. Concerning Ménière's disease, the following are true except:

A. Current American Academy of Otolaryngology–Head and Neck Surgery (AAO-HNS) criteria include possible, probable, definite, and certain diagnostic criteria

B. Aquaporin mutation, saccin regulation, and endolymphatic sac fibrosis are all proposed causative theories in Ménière's disease

C. Lermoyez syndrome represents a variant of Ménière's disease

D. Betahistine has both H1 and H3 receptor effects, altering neurotransmitter levels and causing local cochlear vasodilation

E. Intratympanic gentamicin represents a hearing-preserving option in a patient with serviceable hearing

45. Which of the following statements is false concerning cervical vestibular evoked myogenic potentials (cVEMPs)?

A. They test the otolithic organ

B. The needle is inserted into the ipsilateral sternocleidomastoid

C. Superior semicircular canal dehiscence produces a reduced cVEMP response

D. The test assesses otolithic organ function in the saccule and utricle

E. The test must be performed with the head at a 45-degree angle and the test subject's head raised off the bed

46. The following are tests used in establishing non-organic hearing loss except:

A. Erhardt's

B. Lombard's

C. Chimani–Moos

D. Stenger's

E. Bing's

47. Concerning the internal auditory meatus (IAM), which of the following statements is true?

A. The IAM segment of the facial nerve is 12–13 mm in length

B. The cerebellopontine angle segment of the facial nerve is 8–10 mm in length

C. Bill's bar separates the facial nerve from the cochlear nerve

D. The facial nerve sits anteroinferiorly in the IAM

E. The falciform crest separates the superior and inferior vestibular nerves

48. Sensorineural hearing loss is associated with dystopia canthorum in which syndrome?

A. Pendred

B. Usher

C. Waardenburg

D. Alport

E. Brachio-oto-renal

49. Ewald's first law states that:

A. Nystagmus is generated in the plane of the semicircular canal being stimulated

B. Nystagmus is strongest when gazing in the direction of the fast phase of nystagmus

C. Unilateral weakness may be detected by the presence of nystagmus

D. In the horizontal semicircular canals, ampullofugal endolymph movement causes greater stimulation than ampullopetal endolymph movement

E. Torsional nystagmus is pathognomonic of BPPV

50. A 38-year-old lady describes short bursts of rotatory vertigo associated with head movements and turning over in bed. The Dix–Hallpike test is positive when the head is turned to the left. Which nystagmus would you expect to see?

A. Rotational geotropic nystagmus to the right

B. Rotational geotropic nystagmus to the left

C. Horizontal nystagmus to the left

D. Horizontal nystagmus to the right

E. Upbeating nystagmus

51. With regard to Michel aplasia, which if the following statements is most likely to be true?

A. A relative contraindication for cochlear implantation

B. An absolute contraindication for cochlear implantation

C. An indication for cochlear implantation

D. More common in males

E. Associated with progressive sensorineural hearing loss

52. What is the most appropriate definitive management for 40-year-old windsurfer with recurrent otitis externa and fluctuating moderate conductive hearing loss?

A. Combined approach tympanomastoidectomy

B. Modified radical mastoidectomy

C. Radical mastoidectomy

D. Canalplasty

E. Meatoplasty

53. You are referred a 52-year-old gentleman with a left vagal paraganglioma. Which of the following genetic abnormalities could be associated with this and carries the highest risk of associated malignancy?

A. SDH-A

B. NF-2

C. NF-1

D. SDH-D

E. SDH-B

1. C. The jugular foramen is bordered laterally by the temporal bone but does not enter it.

The internal auditory canal transmits the facial nerve, the vestibular nerve, and the cochlear nerve.

The vestibular aqueduct transmits the endolymphatic duct.

The cochlear aqueduct transmits a prolongation of the dura mater establishing a communication between the perilymphatic space and the subarachnoid space, and transmits a vein from the cochlea to join the internal jugular.

The subarcuate fossa transmits a small vein.

2. A. Koerner's septum is the petrosquamous suture and is the lateral-most limit of the mastoid antrum. In dissection of the temporal bone, therefore, it is opened medial to the mastoid air cells before entering the antrum.

3. B. The cochlear nucleus lies in the brainstem and is responsible for processing sound signals carried from the ear through the vestibulocochlear nerve. Auditory brainstem implants are electrodes placed in the cochlear nucleus.

National Institute for Health and Care Excellence (NICE). *Auditory Brain Stem Implants*. Interventional procedures guidance [IPG 108]. London: NICE, 2005.

4. E. The middle fossa approach involves identifying all structures except the foramen ovale.

5. D. The utricle and the saccule both sense linear acceleration. The utricle senses motion in the horizontal plane (forward–backward or left–right movement), while the saccule senses motions in the sagittal plane (up–down movement).

The superior vestibular nerve is posterosuperior in the internal auditory canal and the facial nerve is anterosuperior.

The inferior vestibular nerve (singular nerve) innervates the posterior semicircular canal. Surgical division of this nerve is used in the treatment of BPPV.

The VEMP reflex is a vestibulocollic reflex whose afferent limb arises in the acoustically stimulable neurons of the saccule. The afferent limb is the inferior vestibular nerve. The efferent limb innervates the ipsilateral sternocleidomastoid muscle.

The main blood supply to the vestibular end organs is from the internal carotid artery via the labyrinthine artery. This usually arises from the anterior cerebellar artery, superior cerebellar artery, or basilar artery. The middle meningeal artery is a branch of the maxillary artery.

6. E. Masking is required for ABR and CER but not ECoG testing.

The ABR is a neurological measure of the brainstem response to an auditory stimulus. ABR testing generates waveform peaks that are labelled I–VII. Wave I represents the action potential generated in the cochlear nerve.

The ECoG is considered to offer poor reliability at low frequencies below 500 Hz. The ECoG has three components: the cochlear microphonic, the summating potential (SP), and the action potential (AP). The SP/AP ratio is used in some centres investigating patients with Ménière's disease. However, an altered ratio is not generally considered to provide an accurate diagnosis.

7. B. There are three times as many outer hair cells than inner hair cells. The majority of the afferent cochlear nerve terminals (95%) synapse on the inner hair cells and transmit sensory signals. Endolymph does have an electrolyte composition similar to intracellular fluid (high potassium and low sodium ions) whereas the composition of the perilymph is similar to that of extracellular fluid (high sodium and low potassium ions).

The stereocilia act as mechanical transducers. Bending of the stereocilia towards the tallest row causes an opening of channels and depolarization. The inner hair cells are arranged in a single row while the outer hair cells are arranged in three rows.

8. C. Angular acceleration is detected by the semicircular canals. The ampullated end of each semicircular canal contains the ampullary crest containing hair cells embedded in the cupula.

When the endolymph moves, the hair cells within the cupula are displaced to one side or the other. Movement of endolymph in the horizontal semicircular canals towards the ampulla (ampullopetal) increases the firing rate, while movement of endolymph away from the ampulla (ampullofugal) results in decreased firing. This is in contrast to the superior and posterior semicircular canals, where ampullopetal flow decreases and ampullofugal flow increases the firing rate.

The horizontal semicircular canals are paired such that increased firing in one canal is balanced by decreased firing in the opposite one.

Thus, when a person is rotated clockwise, the bony labyrinth rotates clockwise while the endolymph remains 'relatively' static due to inertia. This causes the cupula and its hair cells to bend. When the rotation is stopped, the momentum of the now moving endolymph causes it to continue moving. The hair cells are now bent in the opposite direction. Thus, in the right ear, the endolymphatic flow is ampullopetal and ampullofugal in the left ear. Right fast-beating nystagmus then occurs.

9. A. Otoacoustic emissions represent sound generated by the outer hair cells, typically in response to a sound stimulus. The emissions are frequently absent in conductive hearing loss and are usually absent in severe sensorineural hearing loss although they do not exclude an absent cochlear nerve. The testing is objective and is therefore used in the universal neonatal screening programme. Evoked otoacoustic emissions are generated in the majority (approximately 90%) of a normal population.

10. D. Speech audiometry can be useful in patients with probable feigned hearing loss but it cannot always discriminate between the two.

Spondees are bisyllabic words that emphasize both syllables. The speech recognition threshold is the softest level (dB) that an individual can repeat at least 50% of the spondees. The maximal discrimination score is the highest percentage of spondees that an individual can repeat at least 50% of the time. In a conductive deafness, this is likely to remain unchanged but require a louder stimulus.

Roll over describes the phenomenon whereby the speech discrimination score deteriorates with increasing loudness. This can be associated with retrocochlear pathology.

11. E. The decibel scale is calculated based on the $10 \log_{10}$ (Ix/Io) formula, where Ix is the sound intensity being measured and Io is a reference intensity. Each 10 dB increase represents a tenfold increase in the intensity of sound ($\log_{10} 10 = 1$).

The outer hair cells are more susceptible than the inner hair cells. Continuous noise is more damaging than intermittent noise of the same frequency and intensity. Theories concerning noise-induced hearing loss include metabolic exhaustion of the hair cells following the temporary threshold shift that occurs in noise exposure. The hair cells do not regenerate.

12. B. The 2005 Control of Noise at Work Regulations set the lower exposure level at a daily or weekly personal noise exposure of 80 dB (A-weighted) and a peak sound pressure of 135 dB (C-weighted). The upper exposure action values are a daily or weekly personal noise exposure of 85 dB (A-weighted) and a peak sound pressure of 137 dB (C-weighted). At these levels, the employer is required to try to reduce exposure to as low a level as is reasonably practicable by establishing and implementing a programme of organizational and technical measures and provide personal hearing protectors.

13. E. NF2 is an inherited autosomal dominant syndrome. The manifestations result from mutations in the *NF2* gene located on the long arm of chromosome 22. The gene product known as merlin serves as a tumour suppressor. Decreased function or production of this protein results in a predisposition to develop the NF2 phenotypic tumours.

14. A. The presence of active chronic otitis media is considered an absolute contraindication to many while the other responses represent relative contraindications.

15. A. Beta-2 transferrin is not unique to the CSF and is found in perilymph and vitreous humour. The test involves an electrochemical diffusion gradient and requires only a small volume and is not affected by blood contamination. A positive finding of beta-2 transferrin is highly sensitive and specific for a CSF leak.

16. C. If the surgeon is confident that the nerve was not injured in the operation, it is reasonable to allow any local anaesthetic to wear off. If the palsy persists, the packing could be removed from the ear.

17. E. The contents of the jugular foramen include the internal jugular vein, the inferior petrosal sinus, the posterior meningeal artery, the cervical sympathetic chain, and the glossopharyngeal, vagus, and spinal accessory cranial nerves. The hypoglossal nerve is not considered part of the jugular foramen.

18. D. Aspirin typically causes a flat hearing loss and is associated with tinnitus. Typically, hearing improves over 2–3 days and the tinnitus resolves.

19. D. The stapedial artery is the artery of the second branchial arch. When it persists, it is a branch of the internal carotid artery, passing through the arch of the stapes to become the middle meningeal artery. The latter is normally a branch of the external carotid. The absent foramen spinosum is characteristic.

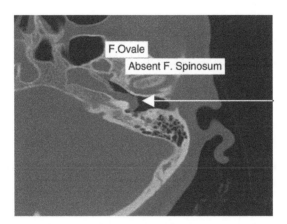

20. D. The axial MRI shows a lesion in the cerebellopontine angle. This is likely to be an acoustic neuroma. Altered sensation of the posterior canal skin (Hitzelberger sign) is due to pressure on the sensory fibres of the seventh cranial nerve carried in the nervus intermedius.

21. E. Hypoplasia of the stria vascularis (Scheibe malformation) is the most common histopathological abnormality found in congenital deafness. This abnormality is found in Jervell–Lange-Nielsen, Refsum, Usher, and Waardenburg syndromes.

Cochlear aplasia (Michel malformation is complete failure of development of the inner ear, both membranous, and bony aplasia) is a severe abnormality and is rare.

Incomplete formation of the bony and membranous labyrinth, such that the middle and apical turns of cochlea occupy common bony space, is a Mondini malformation. This malformation can be seen in Pendred syndrome. This may be asymmetrical and auditory function can vary from normal to profound sensorineural hearing loss.

Dysplasia of the membranous labyrinth with a normal bony labyrinth is known as a Bing–Siebenman malformation.

Partial aplasia of the cochlear duct is the Alexander malformation. This results in high-frequency hearing loss.

22. D. Fluoride ions replace the usual hydroxyl group in hydroxyapatite. The resulting fluorapatite complex is resistant to osteoclastic bone resorption. The recommended dosage varies but is usually 20–40 mg per day. Side effects include rash, arthritis, and gastrointestinal distress. It is thought that hearing can be stabilized in up to 80% of the population.

23. A. A cholesterol granuloma is characterized as having a hyperintense signal character on T1 and T2 MRI imaging and no further enhancement following administration of gadolinium contrast.

24. D. The arcuate eminence is a landmark for the superior semicircular canal.

25. E. In contrast to exostosis of the external ear canal, osteomas are not generally associated with cold water exposure. They are generally considered to be benign tumours and typically contain mature lamellar bone with bone marrow. Surgical removal is usually curative.

26. D. The pinna has a role in localizing sound. The external ear canal acts as a resonant chamber for sounds in the region of 2 kHz. Therefore 'in-the-ear' aids dampen sounds at this frequency. The ratio of the tympanic membrane to the stapes footplate coupled with the amplification of sound through the ossicular lever activity results in an amplification of sound.

27. A. On descent, divers should regularly equalize by performing the Valsalva manoeuvre. However, if this is done too forcibly, the sudden change in middle ear pressure can lead to rupture of either the oval or round window.

28. A. Bell's palsy has an almost universally good prognosis: when paralysis is incomplete (as in House–Brackmann grade IV), function is almost certain to return to normal, whatever intervention is used.

29. B. Gentamicin is particularly toxic to the first row of outer hair cells in the basal turn of the cochlea. Hence patients experience a high-tone sensorineural hearing loss.

30. D. Chordomas are tumours originating from embryonic remnants of the primitive notochord. The tumour occurs in bone, and so they are usually extradural. They can be found in any part of the axial skeleton but occur most commonly in the sacrococcygeus or clivus. Tumours arising in the clivus cause symptoms due to compression and local invasion. This includes headaches and cranial nerve deficits, the commonest of which is the abducent nerve.

Treatment is surgical where possible, with radiotherapy given postoperatively when there is incomplete excision. The tumours are not generally considered to be sensitive to chemotherapy.

31. C. Aminoglycoside ototoxicity usually causes a high-frequency sensorineural hearing loss that is permanent. Damage is usually to the hair cells. Each drug has different effects on the vestibular and cochlear hair cells. Gentamicin is more vestibulotoxic which has encouraged its use in the treatment of Ménière's. Mutations in the 12S mitochondrial rRNA are associated with low-dose aminoglycoside toxicity.

32. B. During ascent, middle ear pressure increases and air can passively pass through the Eustachian tube. In descent, the middle ear pressure reduces and the Eustachian tube, which is normally closed, must be actively opened to equalize pressure. A perilymph fistula can occur due to barotrauma and result in hearing loss and vertigo. Boyle's law states that the volume of a gas is inversely proportional to the pressure at a constant temperature.

33. D. A BAHA may be useful in any cause of conductive hearing loss, including complete absence of the external ear. Learning difficulties are not, in themselves, a contraindication to a BAHA. Patients with a unilateral, but not bilateral, sensorineural hearing loss may benefit from a BAHA.

34. A. Carhart's notch may occur whenever there is a conductive hearing loss. When a bone conductor is applied to the skull, sound reaches the inner ear via the skull and also via the middle ear. This leads to an apparent sensorineural loss when there is a conductive hearing loss. Correction of the middle ear defect results in an apparent improvement in the sensorineural component.

35. A. A visual reinforcement audiogram requires at least two testers and a parent to be present. The child sits a table playing with toys and free-field sounds are produced from a loudspeaker on one or other side of the child. If the child responds to the sound by turning towards it, he/she is 'rewarded' by seeing a visual stimulus (e.g. an illuminated toy jumping in a box); this is the 'visual reinforcement'. The child is then presented with sounds of varying intensities and frequencies and hearing thresholds can be ascertained.

36. C. The standard examination is a T2-weighted series in the coronal and axial planes, followed by a non-echoplanar DWI series (b-values 0, 1000). On the DWI with a b-value of 1000 s/mm^2, a cholesteatoma appears as a hyperintense mass. With a b-value of 0 s/mm^2, the signal intensity will be lower. The ADC map will show low signal in the same region confirming diffusion restriction. Hounsfield units are not that helpful but cholesteatoma will have a Hounsfield unit of 42 ± 24.

37. D. Mumps is not a risk factor for otosclerosis—measles, however, has been shown to have a causal relationship.

38. D. Patients with patulous Eustachian tube complain of autophony and hearing their own respiration. All the other answers can cause pulsatile tinnitus. Carotid dissection is a rare but important diagnosis that should be considered.

39. E. A Mondini malformation of the cochlea results in a cochlea with only 1.5 turns instead of 2.5. Mondini's triad includes an enlarged vestibule but normal semicircular canals and an enlarged vestibular aqueduct. A cochlear implant is appropriate in a Mondini malformation but not with Michel deformity.

40. A. The merlin protein (also known as schwannomin) is coded by the *NF2* gene which is found on chromosome 22 (22q12.2) not 21. The merlin protein functions as a tumour suppressor.

41. E. The tympanic membrane is derived from all three germ cell layers. The inner mucosal surface is a derivative of the first pharyngeal pouch, the intermediate layer from the mesoderm, and the outer layer from the first branchial cleft. Please note the difference between the clefts, pouches, and arches which catch many candidates out.

42. E. The pinna is formed by the 12th week of gestation and will attain its adult shape by the 20th week and be full size by the age of 9 years, which is important when considering unilateral microtia repairs to ensure a match. The lateral one-third of the external auditory meatus (EAM) is cartilaginous and medial two-thirds bony, not to be confused with the Eustachian tube, in which the proportions are reversed. The bony labyrinth develops from 14 ossification centres. Trautman's triangle marks the posterior fossa medially and is a path of infection for extradural abscess formation from ear disease.

43. D. Gradenigo syndrome is caused by petrous apicitis and comprises a triad of diplopia (secondary to cranial nerve VI palsy as it swells within Dorello's canal), retro-orbital pain, and otorrhoea.

44. A. The American Academy guidance of 1995 was revised in 2015 and now includes only probable and definite criteria. Aquaporin mutation, poor saccin regulation, and endolymphatic sac fibrosis are all proposed causes of Ménière's as well as autoimmune causes, membranous labyrinthine microtears, and ischaemic changes, to include but a few. Lermoyez syndrome describes the condition where the common symptoms of Ménière's are relieved by vertigo attacks. Gentamicin is considered primarily vestibulotoxic, contrary to popular belief.

45. C. VEMPs assess otolithic organ function thought to occur due to residual evolutionary hearing potential. The test is performed with sound stimulation and recording either ipsilateral sternocleidomastoid activation (cVEMP) or nystagmus (ocular VEMP). Superior semicircular canal dehiscence produces suprathreshold bone conduction along with increased VEMP activity.

46. C. Bing's test represents a modified Weber's test with a vibrating fork placed over the mastoid process and when it ceases to be heard the examiner's finger is used to occlude the external auditory canal. In normal individuals, the sound will be heard again, indicating a positive test. The remaining tests represent clinical tests which may be utilized to uncover non-organic hearing loss.

47. E. The facial nerve has a cerebellopontine component of 23–24 mm and IAM component of 8–10 mm. The intratemporal component is further subdivided into labyrinthine (3–5 mm), tympanic (12–13 mm), and mastoid (15–20 mm). The cross-sectional orientation of the IAM is separated into superior and inferior sections by the horizontal falciform crest and the superior section further separated by the vertical Bill's bar, which divides the facial nerve anteriorly and superior vestibular nerve posteriorly.

48. C. Waardenburg syndrome is a genetic disorder which can be associated with congenital sensorineural hearing loss. There is a great range of associated symptoms which also vary in severity case to case. The distinctive facial features include diminished pigmentation of the hair, skin, and irides. Dystopia canthorum describes widely spaced eyes, which can be a feature of this syndrome along with a white forelock and heterochromia irides.

Hearing loss associated with Pendred syndrome may be sensorineural or mixed. It is also associated with thyroid goitre and potential hypothyroidism.

Usher syndrome is split into three distinctive types, all of which display varying degrees of sensorineural hearing loss. It is associated with progressive loss of vision.

Alport syndrome is associated with sensorineural, conductive, or mixed hearing loss. Other features can include nephritis, palate abnormalities, myopia, or cataracts.

Hearing loss with brachio-oto-renal syndrome can be conductive, sensorineural, or mixed. It does not have any distinctive ocular signs.

49. A. Ewald was a German physiologist who carried out experimental work in the early twentieth century on vestibular function. He is best known for his description of 'Ewald's three laws':

1. A stimulation of the semicircular canal causes a movement of the eyes in the plane of the stimulated canal.
2. In the horizontal semicircular canals, an ampullopetal endolymph movement cases a greater stimulation than an ampullofugal one.
3. In the vertical semicircular canals, the reverse is true (an ampullofugal endolymph movement cases a greater stimulation than an ampullopetal one.)

Ewald's second and third laws form the basis of the head impulse test which is commonly used today in balance assessment.

50. B. This clinical description is typical of BPPV, which is classically associated with rotational geotropic nystagmus with the affected ear down.

51. B. Michel aplasia is a congenital abnormality of the inner ear. It is characterized by profound sensorineural deafness and complete labyrinthine aplasia. It is therefore an absolute contraindication for cochlear implantation.

52. D. A 40-year-old windsurfer is likely to have developed bony exostoses secondary to exposure to cold sea water. He is getting recurrent infections, which will not be helped, but could be worsened, by a hearing aid, so canalplasty is the optimal management in this situation.

53. E. SDH-B is associated with paragangliomas and a high risk of malignancy.

1. In the course of performing a parotidectomy, you are having difficulty identifying the facial nerve. Which of the following would be least useful in identifying the nerve?
    A. Following the posterior belly of digastric
    B. Identifying the tip of the styloid process
    C. Drilling out the mastoid bone
    D. Following peripheral branches proximally
    E. Following the tympanomastoid suture

2. A patient presents with diplopia and nasal obstruction. He is found to have a nasopharyngeal carcinoma that extends though the foramen lacerum into the cavernous sinus. Which of the following is least likely to be affected?
    A. Oculomotor nerve
    B. Trochlear nerve
    C. Ophthalmic division of the trigeminal nerve
    D. Mandibular division of the trigeminal nerve
    E. Sympathetic plexus

3. Your registrar is performing a total laryngectomy without a neck dissection. As part of the dissection, he has confidently identified the hypoglossal nerve. He then identifies a further nerve, running in the same direction as the hypoglossal nerve but medial to the common carotid artery. What would you advise him to do next?
    A. Preserve the nerve and continue the dissection
    B. Dissect the nerve proximally
    C. Dissect the nerve distally
    D. Divide the nerve and continue the dissection
    E. Consider a primary anastomosis after the resection is complete

4. **A 25-year-old professional opera singer attends the voice clinic as an emergency. During last night's performance, she experienced discomfort in her throat and today says that she is struggling to reach high notes. 70-degree rigid videostroboscopy shows an area of acute haemorrhage on her right vocal cord. What would be the most appropriate advice?**

   A. Advise her to perform tonight, but sing with less effort
   B. Prescribe prednisolone and advise her to continue with tonight's performance
   C. Advise her not to perform tonight and rest the voice
   D. Advise her to cancel the rest of her 3-month tour
   E. Perform an urgent general anaesthetic laryngoscopy and incise and drain the haematoma

5. **A 60-year-old man presents to the 'lump in the neck clinic' with a 5 cm solitary lymph node in the upper right cervical region and an abnormal-looking right tonsil. Assuming this is a squamous cell carcinoma nodal metastasis, p16 positive. what is the 'N' classification, using the TNM system (8th edition)?**

   A. N1
   B. N2
   C. N2a
   D. N2b
   E. N3

6. **A patient presents with a squamous cell carcinoma of the maxillary sinus. Which are the first-echelon nodes for this tumour?**

   A. Intraparotid lymph nodes
   B. Preauricular lymph nodes
   C. Retropharyngeal lymph nodes
   D. Facial nodes
   E. Level III lymph nodes

7. **A patient develops a chylous fistula following a left neck dissection. Which of the following treatments is least likely to result in the fistula closing?**

   A. Endovascular embolization of the thoracic duct
   B. Enteral diet with containing predominantly medium-chain fatty acids
   C. Surgical re-exploration
   D. Enteral diet containing predominantly long-chain fatty acids
   E. Total parenteral nutrition

8. **You see a 46-year-old man with a 3-month history of a mass in the right anterior triangle of his neck. He has smoked 20 cigarettes a day for the last 25 years and drinks in excess of 30 units of alcohol per week. Full ENT examination is otherwise normal. Fine needle aspiration cytology produces 30 mL of milky brown fluid. At 1 week, the cyst has reaccumulated and the cytology reports that the fluid contains cholesterol crystals. What is the most appropriate management?**
   A. Repeat the fine needle aspiration cytology
   B. Reassure the patient and discharge
   C. Commence broad-spectrum antibiotics and review in 6 weeks
   D. Refer the patient to the oncologists for chemoradiotherapy
   E. Arrange for surgical removal of the cyst along with rigid endoscopy of the upper aerodigestive tract

9. **Which of the following statements is most appropriate concerning thyroid cancer?**
   A. Papillary and follicular thyroid carcinomas occur with an equal incidence
   B. Follicular thyroid cancers can be diagnosed using fine needle aspiration cytology (FNAC)
   C. A FNAC report of a solitary thyroid nodule reported as Thy 2 should lead directly on to thyroid surgery
   D. Medullary thyroid carcinoma associated with multiple endocrine neoplasia (MEN) 2B carries a better prognosis than that associated with MEN 2A
   E. Primary medullary thyroid carcinoma does not occur in a thyroglossal cyst

10. **Following enucleation of a superficial pleomorphic adenoma, a patient develops a parotid fistula that discharges onto the cheek. Which is the least effective treatment?**
   A. Repeat aspiration
   B. Compression
   C. Vidian neurectomy
   D. Completion parotidectomy
   E. Tympanic neurectomy

11. **Which of the following statements is true with respect to juvenile nasal angiofibroma?**
   A. It is centred on the sphenopalatine foramen
   B. It rarely recurs after excision
   C. It occurs predominantly in adolescent females
   D. It usually presents with a mass in the neck
   E. It has an association with HLA B17

12. **A 45-year-old lady attends the clinic complaining of dry eyes and mouth. You suspect primary Sjögren syndrome. Which investigation would be most likely to confirm the diagnosis?**

    A. Schirmer's test

    B. Cytoplasmic antineutrophil cytoplasmic antibody (cANCA) testing

    C. ssRho antibody testing

    D. Rheumatoid factor levels

    E. Salivary gland biopsy

13. **You are called to the Accident and Emergency department to see a 46-year-old male who has been stabbed in the neck with a kitchen knife following a domestic dispute. The knife is still in the neck, entering just above the clavicle on the right side. The patient is haemodynamically stable, talking in complete sentences with no respiratory compromise, but is finding swallowing painful. What is the most appropriate next stage of his management?**

    A. Remove the knife and close the wound

    B. Remove the knife and explore the wound in the Accident and Emergency department

    C. Arrange a contrast radiographic swallow examination

    D. Perform an angiogram

    E. Perform a barium swallow

14. **A tumour in the pterygopalatine fossa may have developed there primarily or it may have spread directly into the fossa from any of the following except:**

    A. Orbit through the infraorbital fissure

    B. The cranial cavity through the foramen ovale

    C. The cranial cavity through the foramen rotundum

    D. The nasal cavity

    E. The oral cavity through the greater palatine canal

15. **A 46-year-old man presents with a 5-day history of an upper respiratory tract infection and 2 days' right cervical lymphadenopathy. He is febrile with a raised white cell count. Ultrasonography of his neck reveals a thrombus in his right internal jugular vein and a chest X-ray is reported as having changes consistent with 'septic emboli'. Which is the most likely organism responsible for his symptoms?**

    A. *Proteus mirabilis*

    B. *Clostridium difficile*

    C. *Fusobacterium necrophorum*

    D. *Streptococcus pyogenes*

    E. *Staphylococcus aureus*

16. **A carotid body tumour is likely to receive its major blood supply from which vessel?**
    A. Common carotid artery
    B. Ascending pharyngeal artery
    C. Superior thyroid artery
    D. Lingual artery
    E. Thyrocervical trunk

17. **The registrar calls you in for advice. He is performing a rigid oesophagoscopy on a 38-year-old male with a suspected food bolus obstruction. He has found a smooth, non-pulsatile indentation on the anterior aspect of the oesophagus at 27 cm measured from the upper incisors. The overlying mucosa appears normal. What is this likely to represent?**
    A. The cricopharyngeal sphincter
    B. The left main bronchus
    C. The aorta
    D. The gastro-oesophageal junction
    E. The left atrium

18. **A 46-year-old Caucasian male presents with a postnasal space mass and a 5 cm ipsilateral lymph node. Biopsy of the postnasal space is reported as non-keratinizing squamous cell carcinoma. The most appropriate treatment is:**
    A. Radiotherapy to the postnasal space and ipsilateral modified radical neck dissection
    B. Chemoradiotherapy to the postnasal space, ipsilateral modified radical neck dissection, and contralateral selective neck dissection
    C. Surgical debulking of the postnasal space, bilateral modified radical neck dissections, and postoperative radiotherapy
    D. Primary chemoradiotherapy
    E. Palliative care

19. **Concerning positron emission tomography (PET)-FDG scanning, which of the following statements is true?**
    A. The radioactive tracer is highly specific for cancer cells
    B. PET scanning can define very small tumour deposits of only a few cells
    C. PET scanning has an emerging role in the assessment of the unknown primary
    D. PET scanning can differentiate areas of inflammation and cancer deposits
    E. PET scanning combined with computed tomography (CT) scanning provides improved resolution of the soft tissues compared to magnetic resonance scanning

20. **A patient with medullary thyroid carcinoma is also found to have hyperparathyroidism, and genetic analysis reveals a *RET* proto-oncogene germline mutation. No other physical or biochemical abnormalities are found. What is the most likely diagnosis?**
    A. Multiple endocrine neoplasia 1
    B. Multiple endocrine neoplasia 2A
    C. Multiple endocrine neoplasia 2B
    D. Familial medullary thyroid carcinoma
    E. Sporadic medullary thyroid carcinoma

21. **As part of completing a modified radical neck dissection, you are required to ligate the superior end of the internal jugular vein (IJV). What is the most common relationship to the spinal accessory nerve?**
    A. The jugular vein commonly splits around the spinal accessory nerve
    B. The spinal accessory nerve is medial to the IJV at the skull base
    C. The spinal accessory nerve is lateral to the IJV at the skull base
    D. The spinal accessory nerve has an equal chance of being medial or lateral to the IJV
    E. The spinal accessory nerve is unlikely to be found at the upper end of the IJV

22. **Concerning obstructive sleep apnoea (OSA), which one of the following statements is true?**
    A. During sleep, muscle tension is maximal during rapid eye movement (REM) sleep
    B. The multiple sleep latency test cannot be used to diagnose OSA
    C. Pulse oximetry can accurately diagnose OSA
    D. The respiratory distress index (RDI) is the number of apnoeas/hypopnoeas occurring every hour
    E. Continuous positive airway pressure is unacceptable first-line treatment in a young person

23. **A 24-year-old male HGV driver presents with a history of snoring, day time sleepiness, and obstructive sleep apnoea (OSA), confirmed with a polysomnogram. He is hypertensive, has a body mass index of 30, a neck size of 17 inches, and his respiratory disturbance index is 18. Which of the following statements least accurately describes OSA and its treatment in this patient?**
    A. There may be a direct relationship between his OSA and hypertension
    B. Weight loss is a mainstay of treatment
    C. He should inform the Driver and Vehicle Licensing Agency (DVLA) regarding his condition and cease driving
    D. Uvulopalatopharyngoplasty (UVPP) should be considered as his primary treatment
    E. There is good evidence that treating his OSA will improve his quality of life and reduce his blood pressure

24. **A 44-year-old female professional singer presents with a 3-month history of a swelling in her thyroid gland. An initial fine needle aspiration (FNA) has been reported as Thy 1. A second FNA 6 weeks later under ultrasound (US) guidance is reported as Thy 3. The US reports a 1 cm nodule in the left thyroid lobe. She is biochemically euthyroid and otherwise fit and well. What is the next most appropriate management plan?**

A. Repeat the FNA

B. Reassure her and arrange a repeat follow-up appointment in 3 months

C. Arrange for her to undergo a left hemithyroidectomy

D. Arrange a contract CT scan to exclude a retrosternal goitre

E. Request serum thyroglobulin levels

25. **A 47-year-old woman attends your clinic. She is a heavy smoker and is concerned that her voice is low-pitched and occasionally hoarse. Her larynx has the following appearance. You plan to take her to theatre. What is your first priority in her surgical management?**

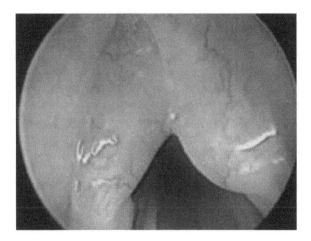

A. Stripping of the vocal cords

B. Incision and drainage of the oedema on one side

C. Incision and drainage of the oedema on both sides

D. Close examination of the post-cricoid region

E. To take biopsies

26. **You are taking consent to proceed with drainage of the oedema in the same 47-year-old woman as in question 25. You explain that you aim to drain the fluid in the vocal cords. Relating to the voice, what affect is this likely to have on her voice?**
    A. She may lose her voice altogether
    B. Her voice may go up in pitch
    C. Her voice may go down in pitch
    D. She should not use her voice for 2 weeks postoperatively
    E. Her singing voice will improve

27. **As part of a multidisciplinary team in a voice clinic, which of the following professionals might you not expect to find present?**
    A. Occupational therapist
    B. Speech and language therapist
    C. Manual therapist
    D. Singing teacher
    E. Psychologist

28. **You are called to see a 44-year-old woman who has undergone a completion thyroidectomy earlier in the day for follicular carcinoma (T2, N0, M0). She is feeling light-headed and short of breath. The foundation year 2 (FY2) hospital at night doctor has checked her serum biochemistry and performed an electrocardiogram (ECG), which is normal. She has been prescribed levothyroxine 20 µg, three times daily. There are no other clinical findings. What is the next most appropriate action?**

Table 3.1 Biochemistry results

Sodium	**137** mmol/L (135–145)
Potassium	**4.4** mmol/L (3.5–5.0)
Urea	**4.9** mmol/L (2.5–6.7)
Creatinine	**89** mmol/L (60–123)
C-reactive protein	**34** mg/L (0–8)
Bilirubin	**8** µmol/L (3–17)
Alanine transaminase	**12** IU/L (10–45)
Alkaline phosphatase	**239** IU/L (110–700)
Albumin	**37** g/L (35–50)
Corrected calcium	**2.20** mmol/L (2.12–2.62)

   A. Start thyroxine (T4) at 100 µg/day
   B. Prescribe calcium gluconate
   C. Prescribe alfacalcidol
   D. Reassure her
   E. Prescribe oral calcium gluconate and recheck the serum biochemistry at 24 hours

29. **Which of the following statements best describes the parapharyngeal space?**

    A. The stylomandibular ligament separates the parapharyngeal space from the submandibular space
    B. The foramen ovale opens directly into the parapharyngeal space
    C. The parapharyngeal space is divided into pre- and post-styloid spaces. The pre-styloid space contains the internal carotid artery
    D. The majority of primary tumours arising in the parapharyngeal space are benign
    E. The pre-styloid space contains the cranial nerves IX–XII

30. **A laryngeal squamous cell carcinoma has spread from the vocal cord into the pre-epiglottic space. For the tumour to continue to spread anteriorly into the subcutaneous tissues and skin, through which structure will it pass?**

    A. Epiglottis
    B. Thyrohyoid ligament
    C. Thyroepiglottic ligament
    D. Aryepiglottic fold
    E. Cricoid cartilage

31. **Concerning the hypopharynx and tumours arising within it, which of the following statements is least likely to be correct?**

    A. The hypopharynx is defined as extending from the superior aspect of the hyoid to the lower border of the cricoid cartilage
    B. Squamous cell carcinomas arising in the post-cricoid region are more common in males
    C. Pooling of saliva in the pyriform fossa may be the only sign of pathology using awake flexible endoscopy
    D. Tumours arising from the pyriform sinus can spread directly into the paraglottic space
    E. A leiomyoma is the commonest benign tumour of the hypopharynx

32. The following diagram is a schematic representation of the vocal fold. In which layer is a patient most likely to develop Reinke's oedema?

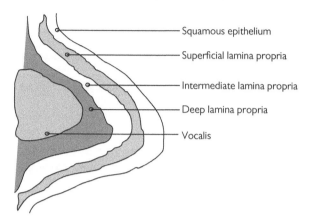

- Squamous epithelium
- Superficial lamina propria
- Intermediate lamina propria
- Deep lamina propria
- Vocalis

A. Squamous epithelium
B. Superficial lamina propria
C. Intermediate lamina propria
D. Deep lamina propria
E. Vocalis

33. A 45-year-old female professional vocalist presents with a solitary right thyroid nodule. She is biochemically euthyroid and a full ENT examination is otherwise normal. A fine needle aspiration is performed and reported as 'possible follicular neoplasm'. What is the next most appropriate action?

A. Reassure the patient and discharge
B. Reassure the patient and review in 6 months
C. Refer for radioactive iodine
D. Screen for a phaeochromocytoma
E. Advise right hemithyroidectomy

34. Which of the following is least likely to be improved following orbital decompression for Graves-associated thyroid eye disease?

A. Optic neuropathy
B. Diplopia
C. Exophthalmos
D. Cosmesis
E. Exposure keratitis

35. **A 46-year-old male presents with left-sided nasal obstruction and a single 5 cm left supraclavicular mass. Biopsy of the postnasal space tumour confirms a diagnosis of non-keratinizing nasopharyngeal carcinoma. According to the Union for International Cancer Control (UICC) TNM (8th edition) grading system, what is the CORRECT stage of neck disease?**

    A. N1
    B. N2
    C. N2a
    D. N2b
    E. N3

36. **A 34-year-old man presents with a mass in the right side of his neck in level 5. He is euthyroid, otherwise asymptomatic, and a full ENT examination is otherwise normal. A fine needle aspiration is performed and this is reported as 'normal thyroid cells'. What is the most appropriate next course of action?**

    A. Reassure the patient and discharge them
    B. Reassure the patient and review in 6 months
    C. Arrange for a lymph node biopsy
    D. Refer them to the thyroid multidisciplinary team for a thyroidectomy and neck dissection
    E. Arrange for radioactive iodine to be administered

37. **A 46-year-old, non-smoker patient presents with a long history of right-sided throat discomfort. He has no dysphagia and full ENT examination is normal. A lateral neck X-ray is requested. What is the most likely cause for his symptoms?**

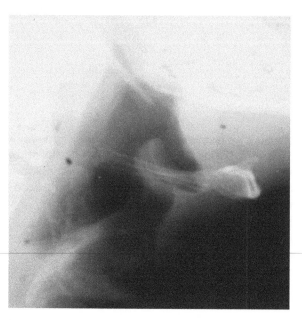

A. Irritation of the vagus nerve
B. Irritation of the glossopharyngeal nerve
C. Irritation of the hypoglossal nerve
D. Irritation of the superior laryngeal nerve
E. Irritation of the cervical plexus

38. **A 65-year-old woman is found to be hypercalcaemic. In locating a parathyroid tumour, which of the following would be the least appropriate imaging modality?**
    A. Ultrasound
    B. Radio-iodine isotope scanning
    C. Magnetic resonance imaging (MRI) scan of the neck
    D. Sestamibi scanning
    E. MRI scan of the chest

39. **Which of the following treatments is least appropriate in the management of medullary thyroid cancer?**
    A. Radiation therapy
    B. Chemotherapy
    C. Radioactive iodine
    D. Surgery
    E. Prophylactic surgery in childhood

40. **You are taking consent from a 25-year-old lady for excision of a second branchial arch cyst. What risks would it be reasonable not to mention?**

    A. Paraesthesia to the ear and neck
    B. Altered tongue movements
    C. Altered facial movements
    D. Altered voice
    E. Numbness to the cheek

41. **You are counselling a 32-year-old woman about thyroidectomy for her Graves' disease. Which of the following statements is true?**

    A. Her eye symptoms and signs are more likely to improve with radio-iodine than surgery
    B. She would be best served by having a subtotal thyroidectomy
    C. Transient hypocalcaemia is very rare
    D. Superior laryngeal nerve injury is usually asymptomatic
    E. Recurrent laryngeal nerve injury is usually asymptomatic

42. **A 72-year-old smoker presents to the ENT clinic with a 3-month history of dysphagia and weight loss. Flexible nasendoscopy shows pooling of saliva in the pyriform fossae, with restricted mobility of the right hemi-larynx. Malignancy is suspected. You proceed to general anaesthetic endoscopy. At surgery, you find that he has a 3 cm tumour affecting the right pyriform fossa and extending into the post-cricoid region. According to the TNM (8th edition), staging, what T stage is this malignancy?**

    A. T1
    B. T2
    C. T2B
    D. T3
    E. T4

43. **A 25-year-old lady presents with a midline neck mass. Clinically and radiographically, it is a thyroglossal duct cyst. It is excised in a Sistrunk's procedure, including the middle one-third of the hyoid bone. Histology shows a papillary carcinoma in the cyst. Review of the radiology shows no masses in the thyroid itself or lymphadenopathy. What would be the most appropriate management of this malignancy?**

    A. External beam radiotherapy
    B. Subtotal thyroidectomy
    C. Total thyroidectomy followed by radio-iodine ablation
    D. Radio-iodine ablation only
    E. Reassure the patient that the cancer has been excised

44. **A 60-year-old man undergoes a laryngectomy and ipsilateral neck dissection for a T3, N1 laryngeal carcinoma. Which of the following would not, on its own, be an indication for postoperative radiotherapy?**

A. Extracapsular spread

B. Multiple involved lymph nodes

C. Multiple levels of nodes affected

D. Maximal lymph node size 3 cm

E. Close excision margins

45. **You have just started a neck dissection on a 55-year-old man with a performance status of 0, co-morbidity score of 1, when the anaesthetist tells you he is worried that the patient is severely hypotensive and tachycardic. What is the next best course of action?**

A. Descrub and call the adult crash team

B. Ask the anaesthetist to administer 0.5 mL of 1 in 10,000 adrenaline via an intramuscular route

C. Ask the anaesthetist to administer a bolus of fluid

D. Stop operating, and be prepared to abandon the procedure

E. Ask for an arterial blood gas test to check whether there has been unexpected blood loss

46. **A 35-year-old female is referred to the on-call ENT team, having eaten a lamb chop the day before, and has had a persistent foreign body sensation on swallowing. The patient is systemically well and observations are normal. The lateral soft tissue X-ray you have arranged is shown. What is the next best course of action?**

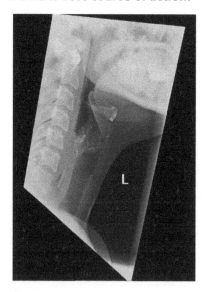

A. Arrange a barium swallow

B. Arrange a MRI neck

C. Plan an oesophagoscopy under general anaesthetic

D. Admit, manage conservatively, and review the next day

E. Reassure and discharge

47. **Which statement is incorrect regarding an individual's risk of developing hypothyroidism?**

    A. The prevalence of spontaneous hypothyroidism is 1%
    B. The risk is ten times greater for women compared to men
    C. Lifetime risk does not change following neck radiotherapy
    D. The commonest cause is chronic lymphocytic thyroiditis
    E. Thyroid autoimmunity is inherited in an autosomal dominant fashion

48. **A 73-year-old woman on warfarin has presented following a mechanical fall. The non-contrast CT head has excluded an intracerebral bleed, but identified an incidental lesion in the parapharyngeal space. You confirm the presence of a smooth mass on nasendoscopy, with no other symptoms or signs. What is the next best course of action?**

    A. Reassure and discharge
    B. List for excision
    C. Ultrasound-guided fine needle aspiration
    D. MRI with contrast
    E. List for panendoscopy and biopsy

49. Following on from question 48, please review the patient's imaging results. What is the most likely diagnosis for this asymptomatic lesion?

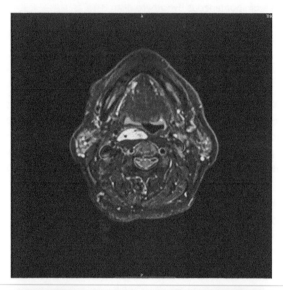

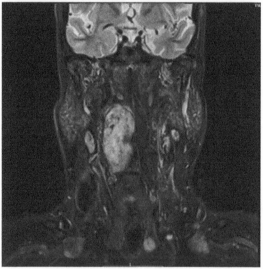

A. Lymphoma

B. Schwannoma

C. Warthin's tumour

D. Metastatic lymph node

E. Lipoma

50. **A 50-year-old non-smoking male presents with a level IIa neck mass measuring 3 cm. He is otherwise asymptomatic; head and neck clinical examination including oral cavity examination and flexible nasendoscopy is otherwise normal. What is the next best investigation?**
   A. Orthopantomogram (OPG)
   B. CT neck and chest
   C. PET-CT
   D. Saliva testing for human papillomavirus (HPV)
   E. Clinical fine needle aspiration of neck mass

51. **The following are side effects of carbimazole except:**
   A. Agranulocytosis
   B. Arthralgia
   C. Jaundice
   D. Hypertrichosis
   E. Taste disturbance

52. **A 45-year-old male with rheumatoid arthritis presents as a 2-week wait patient with a large retromolar oral ulcer. What is the most likely diagnosis?**
   A. Pemphigoid
   B. Candidiasis
   C. Fordyce spots
   D. Methotrexate-related oral ulceration
   E. Adenoid cystic carcinoma

53. **In hyperfractionated radiotherapy, which of the following statements is incorrect?**
   A. Overall treatment time reduced, total dose remains the same
   B. Overall treatment time unchanged, total dose received is increased
   C. Dose per fraction is decreased
   D. Significantly higher locoregional control and survival rates
   E. No significantly higher late side effects

54. **Which of the following statements is incorrect with regard to radiotherapy?**
   A. The maximum dose to the spinal cord is 45 Gy
   B. Ulcerated tumours are most susceptible to radiation treatment
   C. Cells are most radioresistant in the S phase of the cell cycle
   D. A higher dose of radiation is required to kill hypoxic cells
   E. Tumours that are chemosensitive are likely to be radiosensitive

55. You are supervising your registrar performing a selective neck dissection. They inadvertently puncture the internal jugular vein (IJV) in level IV. What is the next best course of action?

A. Contact the on-call cardiothoracic surgeon

B. Isolate and ligate the IJV using transfixion sutures at both ends

C. Cauterize the bleeding point using bipolar diathermy

D. Isolate and suture the site of injury

E. Contact the on-call vascular surgeon

56. Which is not an important step during paramedian mandibulotomy?

A. Pre-plating prior to performing an osteotomy

B. Identification and preservation of the mental foramen

C. Identification of the hypoglossal nerve

D. Leaving some gingival mucosa attached to the mandible

E. Review the preoperative orthopantomogram (OPG) to assess for dental roots

57. Please identify which of the following conditions is not associated with candida infection:

A. Oral stomatitis

B. Median rhomboid glossitis

C. Chronic hyperplastic leucoplakia

D. Denture-related stomatitis

E. Lingual erythema migrans

58. A 30-year-old female presents to the head and neck multidisciplinary team with a rapid increase of a left parotid swelling. She is 18 weeks pregnant. The core biopsy confirms an acinic cell carcinoma. Which of the following management options should the multidisciplinary team recommend?

A. Recommend a parotidectomy once the patient is postpartum

B. Recommend a parotidectomy, and postoperative radiotherapy on an urgent basis

C. Recommend a parotidectomy within the third trimester

D. Recommend a parotidectomy on an urgent basis

E. Recommend intensity-modulated radiation therapy (IMRT)

59. Which of the following recommendations is true regarding prophylactic surgery for *RET* gene mutation carriers?

A. Postoperative treatment with radioiodine ablation may be considered

B. Preoperative calcitonin has no role in decision-making

C. Children with multiple endocrine neoplasia (MEN) 2A should undergo prophylactic thyroidectomy within the first year of life

D. Once surgery has been carried out, treatment with thyroxine at a level to suppress thyroid-stimulating hormone is recommended

E. In an asymptomatic postoperative patient with a serum calcium of 1.9 mM, oral calcium supplementation is sufficient

60. **A 60-year-old gentleman with a 2-month history of a hoarse voice is placed on your operating list for a microlaryngoscopy. He has a heavy smoking history. At surgery, the findings are as shown. Please choose the next best course of action:**

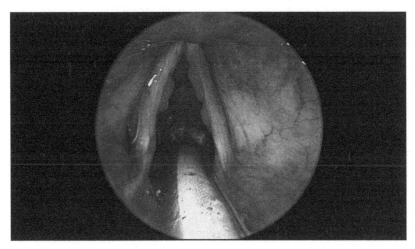

A. Don't biopsy; wake the patient and arrange a CT scan

B. Proceed to biopsy

C. Microdebridement of the lesions

D. CO_2 laser ablation of the lesions

E. Proceed with biopsy; arrange a CT neck and chest and a discussion at the head and neck multidisciplinary team

61. **Which of the following is predictive of permanent hypocalcaemia post thyroidectomy?**

A. Parathyroid hormone level of less than 1.2 at 4 hours postoperatively

B. Calcium less than 2 mM at 72 hours postoperatively

C. Intraoperative parathyroid hormone decrease of greater than 50%

D. Symptomatic hypocalcaemia post surgery

E. Preoperative hypothyroidism

62. **Which of the following tests have concluded a successfully localized overactive parathyroid gland?**

A. A drop in the intraoperative parathyroid hormone monitoring from the pre-skin incision level of 50 pg/mL to 10 pg/mL 10 minutes post removal

B. A difference of 8% between ultrasound-guided right and left internal jugular vein (IJV) serum samples of parathyroid hormone

C. A drop in the intraoperative parathyroid hormone monitoring from the pre-skin incision level of 50 pg/mL to 30 pg/mL 10 minutes post removal

D. A difference of 5% between ultrasound-guided right and left IJV serum samples of parathyroid hormone

E. A drop in the intraoperative parathyroid hormone monitoring from the pre-skin incision level of 50 pg/mL to 30 pg/mL 5 minutes post removal

63. **With regard to spasmodic dysphonia (SD), which statement is false?**

A. Abductor SD is more common

B. Abductor SD is associated with a breathy, effortful voice and abnormal whispered segments

C. The inability to sustain vowels is associated with adductor SD

D. Botulinum toxin is injected into the posterior cricoarytenoid muscle to treat abductor SD

E. Using electromyographic (EMG) guidance, a sniff can indicate correct placement of the needle into the posterior cricoarytenoid muscle

64. **A 53 year old male with a T1N1 (TNM 8) p16 positive scc of the left tonsil is presented and discussed in the head and neck MDT. Following discussion with the patient in clinic, a plan of transoral oropharyngeal resection and ipsilateral neck dissection is planned as the initial mode of treatment. Which best describes your surgical plan?**

A. TORS left oropharyngeal resection, followed by left selective neck dissection including levels 2 to 4.

B. TORS left oropharyngeal resection, followed by left modified radical neck dissection.

C. Left selective neck dissection including levels 2 to 4 and ligation of lingual and facial external carotid vessels, followed by left TORS oropharyngeal resection.

D. Left modified radical neck dissection including ligation of lingual and facial external carotid vessels, followed by left TORS oropharyngeal resection.

E. Left selective neck dissection including levels 2 to 4 and ligation of the facial and maxillary external carotid vessels, followed by left TORS oropharyngeal resection.

65. **The following are adverse features of a thyroid nodule on ultrasound except:**

A. A solid hypoechoic area compared to the thyroid

B. Microcalcification

C. The nodule is described as taller greater than wide

D. Peripheral vascularity

E. Lobulated outline

66. **Please see the figure. The following are all acute radiotherapy side effects except:**

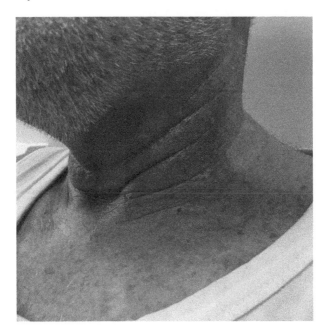

    A. Skin reaction seen in figure

    B. Xerostomia

    C. Otitis media with effusion

    D. Lhermitte's sign

    E. Mucositis

67. **Which of the following statements is true regarding injection thyroplasty?**

    A. It is not indicated in patients with a palliative diagnosis

    B. A possibility of neuropraxia and resultant nerve recovery is an absolute contraindication

    C. It is indicated in patients with a 1–3 mm glottic gap on phonation

    D. Calcium hydroxylapatite is a common short-term injectable preparation

    E. Gelfoam is in common usage for temporary injection thyroplasty

68. **The following are all management options for gustatory sweating following parotidectomy except:**

    A. Sectioning of Jacobson's nerve

    B. Sternocleidomastoid flap

    C. Botulinum toxin injection

    D. Topical deodorant preparation

    E. Temporal fascia flap

69. **With regard to dynamic facial reanimation techniques, which of the following is true?**

A. A gold weight is placed in the suborbicularis plane

B. A sural nerve graft is the most common nerve graft used in cable grafting

C. Following cable grafting, most surgeons aim for a House–Brackmann grade II postoperatively

D. In a nerve to masseter transfer, the nerve is identified 3 cm anterior to the tragus, 1 cm inferior to the zygomatic arch on the surface of the master muscle

E. Temporalis lengthening myoplasty involves detaching the insertion of the temporalis muscle from the coronoid process of the mandible and freeing the temporalis muscle from its posterior aspect to allow reinsertion to the perioral muscles

70. **In a patient presenting with a well-circumscribed T2 squamous cell carcinoma of the left true vocal cord and false cord, a multidisciplinary team recommendation considering all patient factors was to offer surgery. According to the European Laryngological Association Classification for cordectomy, which would be the most appropriate resection to perform for transoral surgical resection of the tumour?**

A. III

B. IV

C. Vd

D. Va

E. Vc

71. **Which of the following laryngeal electromyographic (EMG) findings is incorrectly matched to the diagnosis?**

A. A pattern of decreased frequency and normal amplitude is suggestive of myopathy

B. A picket fence pattern is suggestive of partial reinnervation

C. Fibrillation potentials represent a denervation pattern

D. A fatiguing pattern is suggestive of myasthenia gravis

E. Inappropriate muscle activity in the thyroarytenoid muscle indicates adductor spasmodic dysphonia

72. **A patient is presented at the multidisciplinary team meeting with a history of diabetes, a stroke 12 months ago, and resultant difficulty with feeding and dressing. He now lives in a nursing home. Which is the most appropriate performance status (PS) to attribute to this patient?**

A. PS 0

B. PS 1

C. PS 2

D. PS 3

E. PS 4

73. **Please read the following disease associations and choose the statement least likely to be correct:**

    A. Oral pigmentation and Addison's disease
    B. Oral cobblestoning, lichen planus, and Crohn's disease
    C. Red eyes, oral ulceration, and Stevens–Johnson syndrome
    D. Pyostomatitis vegetans and ulcerative colitis
    E. Recurrent oral vesicles and pemphigus

74. **According to the 8th edition of the American Joint Committee on Cancer (AJCC) cancer staging manual, what stage would be attributed to a patient presenting with a 2.1 cm human papillomavirus-positive squamous cell carcinoma of the left tonsil and a 5 cm left level IIa lymph node metastasis, with no other metastatic disease identified?**

    A. T2, N2a, stage I
    B. T2, N2a, stage IVb
    C. T1, N1, stage I
    D. T1, N2a, stage IVa
    E. T2, N1, stage I

75. **In high-risk human papillomavirus (HPV) infection, carcinogenesis is thought to occur by all of the following statements except:**

    A. The E6 protein binds to the p53 protein
    B. The E7 protein binds to the Rb protein
    C. P53 is a tumour suppressor protein
    D. The degradation of the p53 protein is associated with p16 overexpression
    E. Following binding, the G1 checkpoint is lost

76. **Please choose the most appropriate management option for a patient presenting following narrow excision of a malignant melanoma in the preauricular skin. Histopathology confirms a melanoma measuring 1.1 mm in thickness, with ulceration. There are no enlarged cervical lymph nodes.**

    A. Excise the scar with a 3 cm margin and completion neck dissection
    B. Excise the scar with a 2 cm margin and offer a sentinel lymph node biopsy
    C. Excise the scar with a 1 cm margin and no lymph node management
    D. Excise the scar with a 2 cm margin and completion neck dissection
    E. Excise the scar with a 3 cm margin and offer a sentinel lymph node biopsy

77. **The following are useful assessments to undertake during a modified functional endoscopic assessment of swallow except:**

    A. Assessment of vocal cord mobility
    B. Assessment of laryngeal sensation
    C. Amount of residue noted
    D. Secretion management
    E. Maximum phonatory time

78. **A 75-year-old female presents to your clinic with a longstanding persistent cough. Head and neck examination reveals a fullness of the left aryepiglottic fold, with normal vocal cord movement. Please see the image for assessment at microlaryngoscopy. The most likely diagnosis from the following list is:**

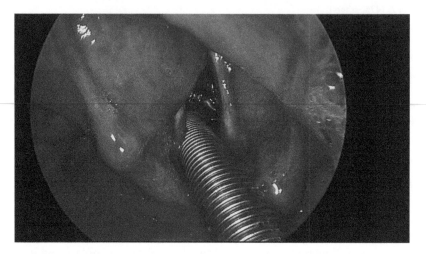

    A. Squamous cell carcinoma of the supraglottis
    B. Internal laryngocele
    C. Mucous retention cyst
    D. Extramedullary plasmacytoma
    E. Bacterial supraglottitis

79. **The following is a list of symptoms and associated diagnoses for dysphagia. Please identify the pair that does not match:**

    A. Reduction of the oral phase of swallowing and Parkinson's disease
    B. A sudden onset of dysphagia in a patient with prior symptoms is suggestive of an oesophageal stricture
    C. Recurrent chest infections with a history of rheumatoid arthritis
    D. Odynophagia and a background of iron deficiency anaemia
    E. Gradual-onset dysphagia worse at the end of day is suggestive of myasthenia gravis

80. **A 45-year-old male patient with a T1 oral cavity squamous cell carcinoma of the lateral tongue measuring 1.5 cm across and 3.4 mm in depth presents to the head and neck multidisciplinary team. The best recommendation based on the information given is:**
    A. Wide local excision and clinical surveillance of the neck
    B. Wide local excision and elective selective neck dissection levels I to III
    C. Wide local excision, radial forearm free-flap reconstruction, and elective selective neck dissection levels I to III
    D. Wide local excision and elective selective neck dissection levels II to IV
    E. Wide local excision, radial forearm free-flap reconstruction, and modified radical neck dissection

81. **A 54-year-old male presents with a T1a mid-cord squamous cell carcinoma. What is the most appropriate treatment to discuss with him?**
    A. Primary cisplatin
    B. Cisplatin-radiotherapy
    C. Transoral laser surgery
    D. Radiotherapy
    E. Cetuximab-radiotherapy

82. **A 46-year-old male presents with a lateral tongue squamous cell carcinoma. In the TNM (8th edition), which of the following factors are not part of the staging process?**
    A. P16 status of the tumour
    B. Size
    C. Size of neck lymph nodes
    D. Number of neck lymph nodes
    E. Depth of invasion

83. **You receive a pathology report stating that the tumour you biopsied is P16 positive. How much of the tumour needs to be positive for the immunohistochemical marker for P16 for the pathologist to report it as positive?**
    A. 100% positivity in malignant cells
    B. More than 90% positivity in malignant cells
    C. More than 80% positivity in malignant cells
    D. More than 70% positivity in malignant cells
    E. More than 60% positivity in malignant cells

84. **A 54-year-old patient presented to the multidisciplinary team (MDT). He has a single 2 cm right level 2 node. This is squamous cell carcinoma on a core biopsy. He is human papillomavirus (HPV)/Epstein-Barr virus (EBV) negative. The patient has undergone a PET-CT scan, panendoscopy, and tonsillectomy. The conclusion of the MDT is that this is an unknown primary. How would this be staged in the TNM (8th edition)?**
    A. Tx, N1
    B. N1
    C. T0, N1
    D. T0, N2a
    E. Tx, N2

85. **Which of the following statements best describes narrow-band imaging (NBI)?**
    A. A radio-isotope study to allow visual inspection of the vascular and mucosal patterns
    B. An optical image-enhancing technology that allows a detailed inspection of vascular and mucosal patterns
    C. A method for treating leucoplakia in clinic
    D. An optical image-enhancing technology that allows a detailed inspection of lymph structures
    E. An optical image-enhancing technology that filters light from cancer cells to produce a void when tumour is present

86. **A 54-year-old man patient presents with a 2 cm right parotid tumour, situated in the superficial lobe of the parotid. Facial nerve function is normal. He has undergone a core biopsy and this is reported as a low-grade mucoepidermoid carcinoma. He has had a PET-CT scan that confirms the parotid tumour. There is no evidence of lymph node or distant spread. What would be the most appropriate initial management?**
    A. Superficial parotidectomy, facial nerve preservation, and level I–IV neck dissection
    B. Superficial parotidectomy, facial nerve preservation, and no neck dissection
    C. Total parotidectomy, facial nerve resection, and level I–IV neck dissection
    D. Primary concurrent chemoradiotherapy
    E. Brachytherapy

87. **When staging a tonsil tumour, which of the following factors will not be used in the TNM (8th edition) classification?**
    A. Size of the tumour
    B. Number of lymph nodes
    C. P16 status
    D. Extracapsular spread
    E. Smoking history

1. B. The tip of the styloid process is variable in position and therefore a poor method for identifying the facial nerve. All of the others are acceptable methods of finding the facial nerve.

2. D. The cavernous sinuses are located at the base of the skull. The internal carotid artery and the sympathetic plexus pass through the sinus. The oculomotor (third), trochlear (fourth), and abducent (sixth) cranial nerves are attached to the lateral wall of the sinus. The ophthalmic and maxillary divisions of the fifth cranial nerve are embedded in the wall. The mandibular division of the trigeminal nerve does not pass through the sinus.

3. D. This is likely to represent the superior laryngeal nerve. The superior laryngeal nerve passes along the pharynx medial to the common carotid artery in a similar direction to the hypoglossal nerve. The hypoglossal nerve is lateral to the common carotid artery.

The superior laryngeal nerve separates from the main trunk of the vagus just outside the jugular foramen; it then passes anteromedially on the thyrohyoid membrane where it is joined by the superior thyroid artery and vein. At approximately this level, the external laryngeal nerve leaves the main trunk and the internal laryngeal nerve enters the thyrohyoid membrane.

This nerve is resected as part of performing a laryngectomy.

4. C. She should be advised not to perform tonight and should be reviewed in a few days. It is not necessary to cancel her engagements several months into the future, but she should be closely followed up to ensure resolution of the haematoma.

5. A. Lymph node metastases from tonsil tumours are classified using the Union for International Cancer Control (UICC) TNM classification (8th edition). There is a different classification depending on p16 status :

- N1: single ipsilateral lymph node less than 6 cm in size
- N2: Contralateral or bilateral lymph node 6 cm or less in size
- N3: any node greater than 6 cm in size.

6. C. The nasal cavity first-echelon nodes are the retropharyngeal lymph nodes.

7. D. The majority of ingested fats are triglycerides with long-chain fatty acids. Long-chain fatty acids are esterified in mucosal cells of the bowel wall and transported into the lymphatic system as chylomicrons.

Middle-chain fatty acids, however, are absorbed directly into the portal system without the formation of chylomicrons, bypassing the lymphatics. Therefore, dietary modifications avoiding long-chain fatty acids are important in the treatment of chylous fistula.

8. **E.** This is likely to be a branchial cyst. Surgical excision is recommended as the cyst has reaccumulated. Cystic degeneration of a metastatic lymph node remains a possibility; therefore, endoscopy of the upper aerodigestive tract should be performed as soon as possible.

9. **E.** Medullary thyroid carcinoma (MTC) arises from the parafollicular cells (C cells) of the thyroid. Embryologically, these are derived from the fifth pharyngeal pouch. The thyroid and hence thyroglossal duct is derived from the third and fourth pharyngeal pouches. Therefore, all malignant types of thyroid cancer can arise in the thyroglossal duct except MTC.

About 80% of thyroid cancers are papillary. Follicular cancer represents 10–15%. FNAC cannot diagnose follicular thyroid cancer.

FNAC results are reported as:

- Thy 1: inadequate
- Thy 2: benign appearance
- Thy 3: follicular lesion
- Thy 4: suspicious of malignancy
- Thy 5: malignant cells.

Therefore, a Thy 2 report may not directly lead on to surgery.

The prognosis of MTC associated with MEN 2B is worse than that associated with all other forms of MTC.

10. **C.** Vidian neurectomy is performed for the treatment of rhinitis. The vidian nerve carries parasympathetic innervation to the pterygopalatine ganglia and hence to the lacrimal gland and the mucous glands of the nose, nasopharynx, and palate.

The parotid receives parasympathetic innervation from the inferior salivary nucleus. The glossopharyngeal nerve conveys these fibres to the tympanic plexus (Jacobson's nerve) and then the lesser petrosal nerve. The postganglionic parasympathetic fibres from the otic ganglion then pass to the parotid gland in the auriculotemporal nerve.

11. **A.** Juvenile nasal angiofibroma (JNAs) typically arise in the sphenopalatine foramen, which they expand. They occur almost entirely in adolescent males and may recur after resection. Nasopharyngeal carcinoma, when seen with HLA B17, is associated with short-term survival.

12. **E.** The diagnosis of Sjögren syndrome can be confirmed by demonstrating periductal fibrosis on biopsy of minor salivary glands. The other tests listed may help to support the diagnosis, but only the biopsy will confirm it.

13. **D.** For penetrating neck injuries, the neck is divided into three zones. Zone 1 extends from the clavicle to the cricoid cartilage, zone 2 lies between the cricoid cartilage and the angle of the mandible, and zone 3 from the angle of the mandible to the base of skull.

The injury described is in zone 1. Penetrating neck injuries in this region have a high risk of damage to the carotid and vertebral vascular tree. Furthermore, injuries in this zone can be difficult to control when bleeding occurs with retraction of vessels into the mediastinum. Therefore, in a haemodynamically stable patient with a high risk of vascular injury, a four-vessel angiography is appropriate.

Other structures that are at risk include nerves traversing the neck including the recurrent laryngeal nerve and the aerodigestive tract. These represent less of an immediate risk to the patient but will need to be treated if damaged.

14. B. The foramen ovale communicates with the infratemporal fossa but not directly with the pterygopalatine fossa. The other formina communicate with the pterygopalatine fossa.

15. C. Lemierre's syndrome is a disease usually caused by the bacterium *Fusobacterium necrophorum*. Typically this affects young, healthy adults. Infection leads to inflammation and thrombosis of the internal jugular vein. Septic emboli cause many of the resulting symptoms.

16. B. The major blood supply is typically from the ascending pharyngeal artery. Multiple small vessels may arise from the carotid artery.

17. B. From the upper incisors, typically the cricopharyngeus is at 15 cm, the aorta 22 cm, the left main bronchus 27 cm, and the gastro-oesophageal junction at 38 cm.

18. D. Surgery has no place in the initial management of nasopharyngeal carcinoma, other than obtaining a tissue diagnosis. High-dose radiotherapy to the primary site and both sides of the neck with or without chemotherapy is the primary treatment, even in the presence of lymph node metastasis. There is good evidence that chemoradiotherapy results in better survival than radiotherapy alone, and is commonly used in advanced disease.

Surgery has a role in patients who relapse with lymph node metastasis following primary treatment.

19. C. Positron emission tomography (PET) is a non-invasive, diagnostic imaging technique for measuring metabolic activity of cells. The PET-FDG scan uses a small amount of radioactive material, FDG (fluorodeoxyglucose), which is concentrated in cells exhibiting high rates of glycolysis. The tracer is therefore not specific to cancer cells and can produce false-positive results when concentrated in tissues that also exhibit high rates of glycolysis, such as inflammatory cells. The resolution of PET is being improved but requires a tumour load greater than a few cells. The advent of PET-CT has improved anatomical localization but not soft tissue resolution.

20. B. About 75% of cases of medullary thyroid carcinoma are sporadic while the remaining are genetically determined. Phaeochromocytomas, frequently bilateral and multiple, occur in MEN 2A and 2B syndromes. Hyperparathyroidism due to multigland disease can develop in MEN 2A but is not seen in MEN 2B.

Characteristic phenotypic abnormalities are seen in MEN 2B and include mucosal neuromas and ganglioneuromas, marfanoid habitus, and cardiac abnormalities. Familial medullary thyroid carcinoma is not associated with endocrine abnormalities. The genetic basis of the familial tumours is missense germline mutations in the *RET* proto-oncogene.

21. C. The most common relationship is for the spinal accessory to be lateral to the IJV at the skull base. Less commonly, the spinal accessory nerve can emerge medial to the IJV and rarely the IJV can split around the nerve.

22. D. During sleep, physiological muscle relaxation is maximal in REM sleep.

The multiple sleep latency test measures the time to fall asleep in a darkened room on several separate occasions across the day following an instruction to fall asleep. An average time of less than 7 minutes is considered to be evidence of pathological sleepiness.

Pulse oximetry is commonly used in the diagnostic testing for OSA. However, a normal oximetry tracing does not exclude OSA, particularly in younger patients who do not desaturate during their apnoea episodes.

Continuous positive airway pressure has been established as the treatment of OSA.

23. D. There is limited evidence that UVPP has a beneficial role in OSA. Palatal surgery can make the subsequent use of continuous positive airway pressure more difficult and it is therefore not a first-line intervention.

Several studies have demonstrated that the presence of OSA is an independent predictor of hypertension, allowing for other compounding factors.

Weight management is considered an important therapeutic treatment for all patients with snoring/OSA.

The DVLA requires that he cease driving. As he has a group 2 licence (heavy goods vehicle (HGV)), driving will be permitted only when satisfactory control of his symptoms have been achieved and confirmed by a specialist.

Current evidence suggests the maximal benefit of treatment is in those patients with a RDI greater than 14 and that this can help reduce daytime sleepiness, quality of life, blood pressure, and mood.

24. C. The initial FNA was reported as Thy 1 (non-diagnostic) and was therefore repeated. The second FNA was reported as Thy 3 (follicular lesion/suspected follicular neoplasm). The majority of patients with a Thy 3 FNA will require surgical removal of the lobe containing the nodule with completion thyroidectomy if malignancy is confirmed by histology. Occasionally, an FNA is reported as Thy 3 due to some suspicious findings but may be Thy 2 or Thy 4. The text of the report should indicate these suspicious and the case discussed at the MDT meeting.

MRI and CT scanning can be useful to delineate the size of the goitre. However, iodinated contrast media should be avoided as this reduces the subsequent radio-iodide uptake by thyroid tissue and therefore can limit the use of I^{131} postoperatively.

Thyroglobulin is used in the surveillance of thyroid cancer following surgery. However, the measurement of thyroglobulin before thyroidectomy has no diagnostic or prognostic value and therefore should not be requested.

25. E. Although you will wish to drain the oedema, and some surgeons would advocate this as part of the procedure, the first priority should be to take biopsies of any suspicious areas to exclude malignancy.

26. B. The fundamental frequency of a person's voice is a function of the mass per unit length and the tension in the vocal cords. If the mass per unit length increases, as in Reinke's oedema, the pitch drops. Drainage of Reinke's oedema is likely to result in a raising of the fundamental frequency of the voice. It is particularly important to warn female patients that their voice may be unrecognizable from its former quality.

27. A. The very minimum requirement for a voice clinic is the presence of an ENT surgeon and a speech and language therapist. In some voice clinics, a manual therapist may attend to address musculoskeletal tension issues, and a psychologist may help with the psychological aspects of dysphonia. A singing teacher may also be of great help in treating professional voice users.

28. D. The corrected calcium is within normal limits. Therefore, no further treatment is required. Hypocalcaemia causes neuromuscular and cardiac abnormalities. The patient may report perioral paraesthesia and in severe cases demonstrate irritability, confusion, hallucinations, or seizures.

Neurological findings include the Chvostek sign and the Trousseau sign, facial tetany, and carpopedal spasm respectively. On an ECG, they may have cardiac dysrhythmias and a prolonged QT interval.

29. D. Most tumours of the parapharyngeal space are metastatic disease or direct extension from adjacent spaces. Primary parapharyngeal space tumours are rare, with the majority being benign (80%). The majority of these are salivary gland neoplasia from the deep lobe of the parotid or minor salivary gland tumours.

The stylomandibular ligament separates the parapharyngeal space from the submandibular space.

The superior boarder of the parapharyngeal space is the temporal bone. The fascia connecting the medial pterygoid plate and the spine of the sphenoid passes medial to the foramen ovale and foramen spinosum and these are not considered part of the space.

The parapharyngeal space is divided into pre- and post-styloid spaces. The pre-styloid space contains the retromandibular portion of the deep lobe of the parotid, minor salivary glands, branches of the trigeminal nerve, the ascending pharyngeal artery, and the pharyngeal venous plexus. The post-styloid space contains the internal carotid artery, internal jugular vein, cranial nerves IX–XII, cervical sympathetic chain, lymph nodes, and glomus bodies.

30. B. The pre-epiglottic space is bounded anteriorly by the thyrohyoid ligament. The posterior boundary is the epiglottis.

31. B. Squamous cell carcinomas arising in the post-cricoid region are associated with iron deficiency anaemia (Plummer–Vinson syndrome (also known as Patterson–Kelly–Brown syndrome)) and are more common in females.

The hypopharynx is divided into the posterior pharyngeal wall, post cricoid, and pyriform sinus.

Pooling of saliva in the pyriform sinus (Chevalier–Jackson sign) is a sign of pathology in the pyriform sinus.

Direct spread of tumours can occur through the aryepiglottic fold into the paraglottic space.

32. B. The original description of the vocal fold was by Hirano, who described five layers: the outer layer of squamous epithelium; the superficial lamina propria, which is also known as 'Reinke's space'; then the intermediate lamina propria, the deep lamina propria, and the vocalis muscle.

Hirano M. Structure and vibratory behaviour of the vocal folds. In Sawashimu T, Cooper F (eds) *Dynamic Aspects of Speech Production*, pp. 13–27. Tokyo: University of Tokyo; 1977.

33. E. A well-differentiated follicular thyroid cancer cannot be differentiated from a benign follicular lesion based on FNAC. Histological diagnosis is required to confirm the diagnosis and therefore most of these cases will require surgical removal of the implicated nodule and discussion at an MDT meeting.

34. B. Orbital decompression is a recognized treatment for thyroid eye disease. Indications for treatment include visual loss due to compressive optic neuropathy, exophthalmos causing cosmetic changes, and exposure keratitis. Diplopia occurring preoperatively or postoperatively is relatively common and may necessitate ocular procedures.

35. E. Neck metastases from nasopharyngeal carcinoma are graded differently from other tumours, as:

> NX Regional lymph nodes cannot be assessed
> N0 No regional lymph node metastasis
> N1 Unilateral metastasis in cervical lymph node(s), 6 cm or less in greatest dimension, above the supraclavicular fossa, and/or unilateral or bilateral retropharyngeal lymph nodes, 6 cm or less in greatest dimension*
> N2 Bilateral metastasis in cervical lymph node(s), 6 cm or less in greatest dimension, above the supraclavicular fossa*
> N3 Metastasis in lymph node)* >6 cm and/or to supraclavicular fossa*
> N3a Greater than 6 cm in dimension
> N3b Extension to the supraclavicular fossa**
> * Note: Midline nodes are considered ipsilateral nodes.

36. D. Thyroid tissue in a lymph node was previously referred to as a lateral aberrant thyroid. This is now recognized as being metastatic well-differentiated papillary thyroid cancer. As such, referral to the MDT and surgery will be required. Interpretation of the FNA is made in the context of accurate clinical information regarding the site and a good-quality aspirate.

37. B. There is an elongated styloid process, also known as Eagle's syndrome. This can cause symptoms attributed to irritation of the glossopharyngeal, trigeminal, facial, and vagus nerves. The symptoms include throat discomfort, a foreign body sensation, and neck pain which may be worse on swallowing.

38. B. Location of parathyroid tissue commonly requires more than one modality. A sestamibi scan combined with ultrasonography will commonly locate a parathyroid adenoma. Radio-iodine isotope scanning is used in the follow-up of thyroid malignancy, and has no role in parathyroid tumours.

39. C. Surgery is the mainstay of treatment for medullary thyroid cancer. Surgery in childhood is used to prophylactically remove the thyroid in those patients with MEN syndrome. While radiotherapy has not been shown to improve survival, it may be used to control local symptoms. Chemotherapy is generally considered ineffective but has been used for progressive symptoms. Radioactive iodine is not used.

Perros P, Boelaert K, Colley S, et al. Guidelines for the management of thyroid cancer, *Clinical Endocrinology*, 2014;81 Suppl 1:1–122.

40. E. Excision of a second branchial arch cleft is usually performed in a skin crease and may require a step incision to follow the tract. The greater auricular nerve is at risk during this incision. As subplatysmal flaps are raised, it is possible to damage the marginal mandibular nerve. As the cyst is followed, this may pass through the bifurcation of the carotid artery, and the superior laryngeal nerve, hypoglossal nerve, and glossopharyngeal nerve can be damaged.

41. D. In all but professional voice users, damage to the superior laryngeal nerve is asymptomatic. However, in singers or other performers, superior laryngeal nerve palsy can be devastating.

42. B. This is a T2 tumour because there is involvement of more than one subsite, but the tumour measures less than 4 cm and there is no fixation of the hemilarynx. The subsites of the hypopharynx are the post-cricoid, the posterior pharyngeal wall, and the pyriform fossa.

T staging of hypopharyngeal cancer:

- T1: tumour limited to one subsite of hypopharynx and 2 cm or less in greatest dimension.
- T2: tumour invades more than one subsite of hypopharynx or an adjacent site, or measures more than 2 cm but not more than 4 cm in greatest dimension, without fixation of hemilarynx.
- T3: tumour more than 4 cm in greatest dimension or with fixation of hemilarynx.
- T4a: tumour invades thyroid/cricoid cartilage, hyoid bone, thyroid gland, oesophagus, or central compartment structure (including strap muscles and subcutaneous fat).
- T4b: tumour invades prevertebral fascia, encases carotid artery, or invades mediastinal structures.

43. C. The incidence of papillary carcinoma arising in a thyroglossal duct cyst is less than 1%. Fine needle aspiration cytology should suggest the diagnosis preoperatively. If it is diagnosed postoperatively, the management should be as for any other well-differentiated thyroid cancer.

44. D. Postoperative radiotherapy should be given to any patient at high risk of locoregional recurrence. All of the options except D should ideally receive radiotherapy.

45. D. During this scenario, the patient has become seriously unwell shortly after induction of anaesthesia. Given the physiological abnormalities, the likely diagnosis is anaphylactic shock. The correct action is to stop operating, and prepare to assist, or abandon the procedure. Exposure of the patient may reveal an urticarial rash. The correct dose of adrenaline for anaphylaxis is 0.5 mL of 1 in 1000 adrenaline intramuscularly.

46. C. The lateral soft tissue radiograph depicts a number of abnormal findings. The cervical spine has lost its lordosis. There is a foreign body of bone density in the upper oesophagus with air trapping around it. Urgent removal by rigid oesophagoscopy is warranted.

Dysphagia and odynophagia are the commonest symptoms of a foreign body, together with a history of ingesting a foreign body. Signs and symptoms of mediastinitis complicating a perforated oesophagus include chest pain, increased respiratory rate, pulse, and temperature.

47. C. The prevalence of spontaneous hypothyroidism is between 1% and 2% in the UK. The risk is greater in older women. Subclinical hypothyroidism is similarly of high incidence, roughly 10% in those over 60 years. Chronic lymphocytic thyroiditis (Hashimoto's thyroiditis) is the commonest cause, with 95% of cases occurring in women.

The most common cause of thyrotoxicosis is Graves' disease, then toxic multinodular goitre. Other causes include an autonomously functioning adenoma or thyroiditis.

British Thyroid Association. *UK Guidelines for the use of Thyroid Function Tests*. July 2006. Available at: https://www.baets.org.uk/wp-content/uploads/2013/02/BTA-Guidelines-on-Thyroid-Function-Tests.pdf.

Slatosky J, Shipton B, Wahba H. Thyroiditis: differential diagnosis and management. *American Family Physician* 2000;61:1047–1052.

48. D. Further investigation is required; a biopsy would be contraindicated without further investigation as this could represent a vascular lesion. Furthermore, it is important to ascertain the position of the internal carotid artery which can be displaced medially before a biopsy is undertaken.

49. B. This is a nerve sheath tumour. Nerve sheath tumours are rare, within the parapharyngeal space they are associated most often with the vagus nerve followed by the sympathetic chain. Schwannomas are the most likely histopathological diagnosis, followed by neurofibroma. They are commonly benign, slow growing, and asymptomatic. Symptoms such as dysphagia and a feeling of a mass in the throat have been reported. Treatment is conservative or excision of the lesion. Malignant tumours are reported and serial imaging is recommended with conservative management to track any changes. There is some evidence that PET-CT can distinguish between benign and malignant lesions.

50. C. Workup of an unknown primary is a common topic in the FRCS. Although this neck mass could be a branchial cyst, a PET-CT scan is the most useful test to try and identify a primary in the upper aerodigestive tract. An ultrasound-guided FNA would be more useful than a clinical FNA in what is likely to be a cystic mass/lymph node to identify a solid component. The 2016 NICE guidelines advise a PET-CT scan early in the pathway.

National Institute for Health and Care Excellence (NICE). *Cancer of the Upper Aerodigestive Tract: Assessment and Management in People Aged 16 and Over.* February 2016. Available at: https://www.nice.org.uk/guidance/ng36.

51. D. Carbimazole is associated with bone marrow suppression, including pancytopenia, agranulocytosis, and neutropenia. Gastrointestinal upset and alopecia are other side effects.

52. D. Persistent oral ulceration requires a biopsy to exclude malignancy (most commonly squamous cell carcinoma). Oral ulceration is a common side effect of methotrexate. Fordyce spots, although more common in patients with rheumatoid disease, are small, raised, yellow spots on the buccal mucosa rather than an ulcer. They are sebaceous lipid-containing glands.

Pemphigoid is associated with blistering, compared to pemphigus, which is more commonly associated with ulceration.

53. A. Several altered fractionation methods have been investigated with regard to head and neck cancer. In hyperfractionation, a large number of fractions, with a reduced dose, are delivered in a conventional treatment time to effect a greater overall dose.

This is in contrast to accelerated fractionation in which a larger dose is given per fraction, over a shorter time period. This is with the aim of reducing tumour repopulation between fractions.

Baujat B, Bourhis J, Blanchard P, et al. Hyperfractionated or accelerated radiotherapy for head and neck cancer. *Cochrane Database of Systematic Reviews* 2010;12:CD002026.

54. B. Exophytic tumours are most susceptible to radiation therapy. Tumours are most susceptible in the G2 and M phases of the cell cycle.

Hypoxic cells are less radiosensitive as free radical formation requires oxygen. The dose of radiation necessary to kill hypoxic cells is 2.5–3.0 times greater than well-oxygenated cells. A nice summary of this is by Yip and Alonzi (2013). Similar trials are ongoing in head and neck cancer.

Yip K, Alonzi R. Carbogen gas and radiotherapy outcomes in prostate cancer. *Therapeutic Advances in Urology* 2013;5:25–34.

55. D. A small puncture to the IJV can be identified and sutured (using 5.0 Prolene) or Ligaclips placed to secure haemostasis. It is important to communicate the problem and your management to the anaesthetist and scrub nurse.

Bipolar diathermy is unlikely to be successful in cauterizing an injured area to the IJV.

A more significant injury, or tumour invasion, may require ligation of the IJV, which is best managed with a transfixion suture to ensure it does not slip off.

56. C. Pre-plating reduces malocclusion and malunion; avoiding the mental foramen reduces postoperative numbness. Leaving gingiva attached allows water-tight suture placement post excision. Inadvertently placing a screw into a dental root can result in a non-vital tooth.

57. E. Lingual erythema migrans, otherwise known as geographical tongue, is a benign inflammatory condition thought to be genetic in origin. It is recommended that you check the patient's haematinics and zinc levels. Otherwise, conservative management is indicated.

Oral stomatitis can be associated with denture-related stomatitis. Additionally, it is associated with malabsorption, or immune deficiency, for example, with Down syndrome, HIV, and diabetes.

Median rhomboid glossitis is a local susceptibility to candida. It is associated with denture-wearing, smoking, HIV, and diabetes. A biopsy may be indicated; it has rarely been associated with squamous cell carcinoma.

Denture-related stomatitis usually affects the hard palate and alveolar ridge of the maxilla. Treatment of the candida and improved hygiene of the plate with an antifungal wash such as chlorhexidine usually effects a remedy.

Chronic hyperplastic leucoplakia requires a biopsy as it is more likely to be associated with malignancy.

58. D. The patient is currently in her second trimester, the safest time to operate within a pregnancy. The greatest risk of operating during the first trimester is miscarriage. Operating during the third trimester carries an increased risk of preterm labour and anaesthetic risks. Surgery is the best course of action. It is not safe to offer radiotherapy during pregnancy. Despite the likely low grade of the tumour, treatment should not wait until the end of the pregnancy.

Short J. *Pregnancy Testing Guidance. Risks Associated with Anaesthesia and Surgery in Early Pregnancy.* Royal College of Paediatrics and Child Health. Available at: https://www.rcpch.ac.uk/sites/default/files/Review_of_risk_of_anaesthesia.pdf.

Walton NKD, Melachuri VK. Anaesthesia for non-obstetric surgery during pregnancy. *Continuing Education in Anaesthesia, Critical Care & Pain* 2006;6:83–85.

59. E. Basal calcitonin levels indicate progression to medullary thyroid carcinoma and/or the presence of lymph node metastasis. This can guide the decision to offer a prophylactic neck dissection. Radio-iodine ablation is not used in medullary carcinoma.

Children with MEN 3 (2B) should undergo prophylactic thyroidectomy, certainly within the first year of life but ideally within the first 6 months. In MEN 2A, this can be delayed, depending on the mutation and calcitonin levels to within the first 5 years, or even beyond.

Postoperative thyroxine management should be to keep the thyroid-stimulating hormone concentration at a normal level.

If the patient is symptomatic of hypocalcaemia, or in severe hypocalcaemia (<1.9 mM), intravenous calcium gluconate follow by an infusion is recommended.

Perros P, Boelaert K, Colley S, et al. Guidelines for the management of thyroid cancer, *Clinical Endocrinology*, 2014;81 Suppl 1:1–122.

60. B. A biopsy is mandatory to exclude malignant disease; however, the lesions are confirmed to be respiratory papillomatosis as expected. The patient should be counselled to stop smoking.

61. A. Because the half-life of parathyroid hormone is short, only 3–5 minutes, a low parathyroid hormone level shortly postoperatively is indicative of the need for long-term calcium supplementation. Intraoperative parathyroid hormone measurement is not routinely indicated in thyroidectomy in the UK. Its use has been tested, however, and a less than 70% decline in intraoperative parathyroid hormone measurement together with an absolute value of greater than 15 pg/mL is predictive of normocalcaemia.

A serum calcium level of less than 2 mM after 24 hours, rather than 72 hours after surgery, is predictive of those requiring calcium replacement postoperatively.

Untreated Graves' disease patients undergoing surgery are more likely to have lower serum calcium levels postoperatively, due to injury to the parathyroid blood supply and hungry bone syndrome. This risk can be reduced with preoperative calcium supplementation.

Oltmann S, Brekke AV, Schneider DF, et al. Preventing postoperative hypocalcemia in Graves' patients: a prospective study. *Annals of Surgical Oncology* 2015;22:952–958.

Roh JL, Park CI. Intraoperative parathyroid hormone assay for management of patients undergoing total thyroidectomy. *Head & Neck* 2006;28:990–997.

Solorzano CC, Carneiro-Pia DM. *Intraoperative Parathyroid Hormone Assays*. UpToDate; March 2019. Available at: https://www.uptodate.com/contents/intraoperative-parathyroid-hormone-assays.

62. A. Intraoperative parathyroid hormone monitoring can be used to reduce the risk of bilateral neck exploration when a hyperfunctioning parathyroid gland cannot be localized prior to surgery. There are a number of protocols used to analyse the results. One, known as the dual criteria, requires a sample to be taken prior to incision, but after induction of anaesthesia. The second sample should be taken from the same site 10 minutes after excision. A decrease of greater than 50% and less than the upper limit of the normal range is considered significant, and the surgery concluded.

Ultrasound-guided bilateral IJV measurement can be used to lateralize an overactive gland. A difference of 10% or more is diagnostic.

63. A. Adductor SD is more common, it represents 80% of cases. SD is familial in 12% of cases. The thyroarytenoid and lateral cricoarytenoid muscles are involved in adductor SD. The posterior cricoarytenoid muscle is involved in abductor SD. Adductor dysphonia is characterized by a harsh, strained voice with inappropriate pitch breaks and glottal fry.

64. C. There is evidence to suggest a reduction in the severity of post operative haemorrhage in transoral oropharyngeal resection following ligation of external carotid artery branches. The branches most commonly ligated are lingual and facial, and less frequently ascending pharyngeal.

Ku bik et al. Effect of transcervical arterial ligation on the severity of postoperative haemorrhage after transoral robotic surgery. Head Neck. 2017 Aug; 39(8): 1510-1515.

Gleys teen et al. The impact of prophylactic external carotid artery ligation on postoperative bleeding after transoral robotic surgery (TORS) for oropharyngeal squamous cell carcinoma. Oral Oncology, Volume 72, September 2017, Pages 190-191

65. D. All of the other options as well as intranodular vascularity, globular calcification, and associated lymphadenopathy are suspicious features. Peripheral vascularity is a benign feature. Ultrasound features are classified by a U grading from U1 (normal) to U5 (malignant).

66. D. Lhermitte's sign is an electric shock sensation felt from the nape of the neck to the tips of the limbs on flexing the neck. It usually develops a few months after radiotherapy and is self-limiting.

The acute skin reaction in the photograph was taken 1 week after completion of radiotherapy for early laryngeal carcinoma.

67. C. Injection thyroplasty is a useful technique on its own, or in conjunction with laryngeal framework surgery to improve phonation. Its uses include those patients not suitable for a general anaesthetic, and those managed palliatively to improve quality of life and reduce aspiration risk. The technique can be performed in the office setting, under local anaesthetic.

Calcium hydroxylapatite (Radiesse Voice) is present for between 12 and 24 months post injection. Gelfoam is not in common usage as it requires a large-gauge needle for injection.

68. D. An antiperspirant can be used topically to reduce the symptoms of Frey's syndrome, gustatory sweating following parotid surgery. Jacobson's nerve is a branch of the glossopharyngeal nerve which supplies parasympathetic secretomotor fibres to the lesser petrosal nerve. This supplies the parotid gland via the auriculotemporal nerve.

69. E. A gold weight is a static measure to improve eye closure following facial nerve paralysis. The weight is placed between the orbicularis and the tarsal plate.

Although a sural nerve is superior in length, the great auricular is more commonly used for cable grafting due to its close location, and being well matched for size.

A House–Brackmann grade III is the best achievable result following cable grafting.

The nerve to the masseter is located within the muscle body of the masseter. The other parameters are correct.

70. A. Vd is an extended cordectomy involving the ventricle, Va includes the anterior commissure and anterior contralateral cord, Vb includes the arytenoid, and Vc includes resection of the subglottis.

Remacle M, Eckel HE, Antonelli A, et al. Endoscopic cordectomy. A proposal for a classification by the Working Committee, European Laryngological Society. *European Archives of Otorhinolaryngology* 2000;257:227–231.

71. A. A pattern of decreased frequency and normal amplitude is suggestive of neuropathy, in contrast to decreased amplitude with normal frequency indicating a myopathy.

A picket fence pattern represents polyphasic action potentials with increased parameters, indicating reinnervation.

In contrast, a deinnervation pattern includes fibrillation potentials and complex repetitive discharges.

72. D. The World Health Organization (WHO) PS is used in patients with cancer to assess prognosis and determine the best treatment plan for the patient. It is based on an ability to perform activities of daily living including bathing, dressing, and eating.

PS 0 is a patient who is unlimited in normal activity. PS 1 is a patient who is symptomatic with normal activity, but self-caring. PS 2 is someone who is ambulatory more than 50% of the time, and who may require some assistance for self-care. PS 3 indicates the patients is ambulatory 50% of the time or less, and requires specialist nursing care. PS 4 indicates the patient is bedridden.

West HJ, Jin JO. Performance status in patients with cancer. *JAMA Oncology* 2015;1:998

73. E. The lips are the most common site of Crohn's disease affecting the oral cavity, and can include tags. A cobblestoned appearance is associated with Crohn's disease, which includes mucosal-coloured plaques on the buccal mucosa. These findings are pathognomonic for the disease, and can be used to monitor disease activity. Lichen planus can be associated with both Crohn's disease and ulcerative colitis.

Although oral lesions are more common in Crohn's disease than ulcerative colitis, oral lesions are still associated with the condition, and can similarly be used to monitor disease flare-ups. Pyostomatitis vegetans are small, white pustules with an erythematous base, occurring in the oral vestibule. They can occur in either condition.

The blisters are rarely observed in pemphigus as they are superficial, and easily burst. However, a positive Nikolsky sign is when a blister is formed on rubbing the mucosa.

Lankarani KB, Sivandzadeh GR, Hassanpour S. Oral manifestation in inflammatory bowel disease: a review. *World Journal of Gastroenterology* 2013;19:8571–8579.

74. E. Due to the better prognosis afforded to HPV-positive squamous cell carcinoma of the oropharynx, this has been reflected in the new 8th edition of the AJCC TNM staging of the head and neck manual. HPV-positive oropharyngeal squamous cell carcinoma is classified differently to HPV-negative disease. This distinction is described as those tumours with an overexpression of p16 (≥75%) and at least moderate staining intensity.

In the new classification, the nodal staging is N2 for bilateral or contralateral disease if all lymph nodes are 6 cm or smaller and N3 if the lymph node is over 6 cm.

This same patient would be classified as T2, N2a, stage IVa in the 7th edition of the TNM.

Lydiatt WM, Patel SG, O'Sullivan B, et al. Head and neck cancers—major changes in the American Joint Committee on Cancer eighth edition cancer staging manual. *CA: A Cancer Journal for Clinicians* 2017;67:122–137.

75. D. High-risk HPV types are bound to both *p53* and *Rb* tumour suppressor genes. The E6 and E7 HPV proteins bind to *p53* and *Rb* respectively. Following this, the tumour suppressor proteins are marked for degradation. Following tumour suppressor degradation, the G1 and G2 checkpoints in the cell cycle are lost. In addition to many other processes, Rb is less able to suppress enzymes for gene replication, stimulating cell division.

Degradation of the Rb protein, rather than the p53 protein, leads to p16 overexpression, which has been identified as a sensitive test for HPV in oropharyngeal squamous cell carcinoma.

Chai RC, Lambie D, Verma M, et al. Current trends in the etiology and diagnosis of HPV-related head and neck cancers. *Cancer Medicine* 2015;4:596–607.

76. B. This is stage IIA disease, as the tumour is between 1 and 2 mm with ulceration.

The recommended clinical excision margins are at least 0.5 cm in stage 0 disease, 1 cm in stage I disease, and 2 cm in stage II disease, according to NICE guidelines.

Risk factors for lymph node metastasis include ulceration and Breslow thickness of at least 0.75 mm.

Indications for sentinel lymph node biopsy include stages IB–IIC, with a Breslow thickness of greater than 1 mm. For those tumours in stages IIIB–IIIC, or with positive lymph node metastasis, lymph node dissection is recommended.

Contraindications for sentinel node biopsy include pregnancy, confirmed metastatic lymph nodes, or abnormal lymph drainage patterns, such as relevant previous surgery.

Methods for sentinel lymph node localization include a preoperative lymphoscintigram, which involves injecting a technetium-radiolabelled tracer (such as albumin) into the site of the primary tumour, followed by imaging and marking by the nuclear medical physician. Immediately preoperatively, a blue dye such as Patent Blue V is injected into the primary tumour site. Finally, a gamma probe is used to measure radioactivity in the lymph node.

Marsden JR, Newton-Bishop JA, Burrows L, et al. Revised UK guidelines for the management of cutaneous melanoma 2010. *British Journal of Dermatology* 2010;163:238–256.

National Institute for Health and Care Excellence (NICE). *Melanoma: Assessment and Management.* July 2015. Available at: https://www.nice.org.uk/guidance/NG14.

77. E. A functional assessment of swallow can produce useful information. Overall assessment, including vocal cord mobility, secretion management, and laryngeal inlet sensation, is useful. Base of tongue retraction and laryngeal elevation, and assessment of swallow for different textures is also useful. It is possible to assess usefulness of manoeuvres such as a chin tuck, or head turn in a dynamic test such as an endoscopic evaluation of swallowing (FEES). In addition, it can be useful if biofeedback is needed to improve technique, or compliance.

78. B. This is an internal laryngocele. Risk factors include a chronic cough or repeated Valsalva manoeuvre such as in trumpet playing. It is important to exclude a squamous cell carcinoma which could be obstructing the saccule.

A CT scan is useful and usually demonstrates air or fluid within the cyst. It can also be used to classify the laryngocele and guide operative management. Laryngoceles are classified into internal, mixed, or external in terms of their relationship to the thyrohyoid membrane. Internal laryngoceles are usually endoscopically deroofed or excised often with CO_2 LASER, taking care to avoid or ligate the superior laryngeal artery. Mixed or external laryngoceles are better addressed with external excision via a neck incision.

The image and clinical history do not fit with an acute infection.

A mucous retention cyst is usually more superficial.

This is a typical location for a laryngocoele; a plasmacytoma is a rare entity. In the head and neck, the more common site is the nasal cavity, sinuses, or nasopharynx. Their appearance is often more red compared to the surrounding mucosa.

79. A. In general, a prolonged oral phase of swallowing is noted in Parkinson's disease with a symptom known as 'tongue pumping' (an ineffective extrusion and retraction of the tongue) being pathognomonic for the disease. A delayed pharyngeal phase is also recognized. Although xerostomia is a recognized side effect of levodopa, often patients exhibit drooling due to abnormal neck positioning and reduced spontaneous swallowing.

A sudden onset of dysphagia may indicate a food bolus. A barium swallow should be performed with recurrent symptoms to exclude a stricture.

Cricoarytenoid joint arthritis can cause fixation and resultant aspiration.

In patients presenting with odynophagia, particularly in association with iron deficiency anaemia, a hypopharyngeal malignancy should be excluded with direct visualization.

80. B. In the study by D'Cruz et al. (2015), the first 500 patients were analysed and the trial ended early due to ethical considerations. A clear, statistically significant advantage of overall survival and disease-free survival was demonstrated in the elective neck dissection arm which was performed at the time of primary tumour resection. Prior to this publication, a tumour depth of 4 mm or greater was used as an indication for an elective neck dissection.

However, depth of tumour invasion (different to tumour thickness) is considered predictive of prognosis and has been incorporated into the 8th AJCC TNM classification for head and neck. These will be classified into 5 mm or less; greater than 5 mm up to 10 mm; or greater than 10 mm. Each increase in 5 mm of depth of invasion will increase the T stage by one level.

An alternative option for the patient presented is sentinel lymph node biopsy. This is a newer adoption compared to its use in melanoma; however, it is part of the most recent NICE guideline (2016) to offer it to patients with a T1, or T2, N0 oral cavity squamous cell carcinoma, who do not require free flap reconstruction.

D'Cruz A K, Vaish R, Kapre N. Elective versus therapeutic neck dissection in node negative oral cancer. *New England Journal of Medicine* 2015;373:521–529.

National Institute for Health and Care Excellence (NICE). *Cancer of the Upper Aerodigestive Tract: Assessment and Management in People Aged 16 and Over.* February 2016. Available at: https://www.nice.org.uk/guidance/ng36.

81. C. While both transoral laser surgery and radiotherapy have similar cure rates, the NICE 2016 guideline recommends offering primary transoral surgery for these lesions. However, it would be anticipated that both radiotherapy and surgery options be discussed and the patient's own considerations included in the decision-making.

National Institute for Health and Care Excellence (NICE). *Cancer of the Upper Aerodigestive Tract: Assessment and Management in People Aged 16 and Over.* February 2016. Available at: https://www.nice.org.uk/guidance/ng36.

82. A. In the TNM (8th edition) for oral cavity tumours, size, neck nodal status, and depth of invasion form part of the staging process. P16 status is used importantly for oropharyngeal tumours not oral cavity tumours.

83. D. The Royal College of Pathologists dataset for reporting mucosal malignancies of the pharynx require p16 positivity in greater than 70% of malignant cells.

84. B. The TNM (8th edition) has eliminated the T0 category for tumours that are HPV/EBV negative. This is because an anatomical site cannot be identified. It has retained T0 for neck nodes that are positive for HPV or EBV. In these situations, the tumour would be T0, N1 oropharyngeal tumour if HPV positive or T0, N1 nasopharyngeal tumour if HPV positive.

85. B. NBI is a new technique that filters the illuminating white light on the endoscope into two colours (blue and green), which are avidly absorbed by blood vessels to allow for better visualization of the mucosa.

86. B. ENT UK guidelines published in 2016 advocate preserving the facial nerve when possible. The guidelines suggest that a neck dissection is considered in those with N+ disease or high-risk histology and/or high-grade tumours. The size of the primary tumour is also reported to be important in some series. Primary radiotherapy could be considered by the MDT but concurrent chemoradiotherapy does not have a role.

87. E. In the TNM (8th edition), p16 status is now important. Extracapsular spread is reported for p16-negative tumours only. While smoking has been shown to be important in stratifying prognosis, it is not included in the TNM (8th edition) classification.

1. **A 3-year-old child presents with a discharging sinus below the pinna. On closer inspection, you notice a sinus opening in the external auditory canal. What would be the next appropriate step?**
    A. Proceed to excision, excising an ellipse of skin and removing the whole tract
    B. Arrange a fistulogram to assess the course of the fistula
    C. Arrange an ultrasound scan
    D. Refer the child to the paediatricians because they may have multiple anomalies
    E. Arrange a magnetic resonance imaging (MRI) scan

2. **Which of the following muscles is the most important in opening of the Eustachian tube?**
    A. Levator veli palatini
    B. Tensor veli palatini
    C. Salpingopharyngeus
    D. Buccinator
    E. Lateral pterygoid

3. **A 6-month-old child is being followed up with laryngomalacia having being diagnosed following a microlaryngoscopy and bronchoscopy. In which of the following situations would you consider surgical intervention?**
    A. Noisy breathing during feeding
    B. Cyanotic episodes
    C. Failure to thrive
    D. A and B
    E. B or C

4. **You are called to see a 3-day-old baby born to a lady of Afro-Caribbean descent. The child was born full term in the breech position by vaginal delivery. The child has a firm palpable mass in the region of the right sternocleidomastoid muscle. What is the most appropriate management?**
   A. Fine needle aspiration cytology
   B. Massage and observation
   C. Surgical exploration
   D. Commence antituberculous therapy
   E. Intralesional sclerosant injections

5. **You are working in London and are asked to consent a child born on 24 January 2017 for a tonsillectomy following persistent episodes of tonsillitis. His biological father accompanies him. The father informs you that he has a different surname from his son and has never been married to the child's mother although he is named on the birth certificate as the father. The father wants the operation to proceed. What is the most appropriate course of action?**
   A. Inform the father that only the mother can consent for treatment and therefore postpone surgery
   B. Cancel surgery and see if the child has any further episodes of tonsillitis in the next 6 months
   C. Allow the father to sign the consent form and proceed with surgery
   D. Alter the order of the list so that the hospital lawyer can be contacted
   E. Get a colleague to witness the consent

6. **Which of the following statements best describes the development of the ear in an otherwise healthy child?**
   A. At birth, the ossicles are approximately half their eventual adult size
   B. The auricle develops from the ectoderm of the first three branchial arches
   C. At birth, the auricle is of adult shape and size
   D. The first otological structure to develop is the inner ear
   E. The bony labyrinth develops from six separate centres of ossification

7. **A child presents with a normal auricle, complete external ear canal atresia, and normal middle ear and ossicles. What is the likely timing of the insult that would have caused these changes?**
   A. 0–15 weeks' gestation
   B. 15–25 weeks' gestation
   C. 25–40 weeks' gestation
   D. Postnatal
   E. It is not possible to predict the timing

8. **A 3-year-old child (10 kg) presents to the Accident and Emergency department with a post-tonsillectomy haemorrhage. The child is crying, has a heart rate of 140 beats per minute, and has a normal blood pressure (110/60 mmHg). Up to what volume of blood are they likely to have lost?**

    A. 50 mL
    B. 120 mL
    C. 175 mL
    D. 200 mL
    E. 235 mL

9. **Which subtypes of human papillomavirus (HPV) are associated with recurrent respiratory papillomatosis?**

    A. 11 and 16
    B. 6 and 16
    C. 6 and 11
    D. 16 and 18
    E. 6, 11, 16, and 18

10. **Vaccination against the human papillomavirus (HPV) has been introduced in to the UK to prevent cervical cancer. The vaccine Gardasil offers protection against which strains of HPV?**

    A. 11 and 16
    B. 6 and 16
    C. 6 and 11
    D. 16 and 18
    E. 6, 11, 16, and 18

11. **You are referred a child with congenital hearing loss and a goitre. A diagnosis of Pendred syndrome is made. Which of the following statements is least likely to be true?**

    A. Pendred syndrome is a common form of syndromal deafness
    B. A computed tomography (CT) scan of the auditory system may show a Mondini malformation
    C. A CT scan of the auditory system may show a large vestibular aqueduct
    D. Pendred syndrome is diagnosed when there is a decrease in radioactive iodide discharge from the thyroid following the administration of potassium perchlorate
    E. The chance of a further child being born with the condition to the same parents is 50%

12. **A 14-year-old boy presents to the hospital accompanied by his father with hypovolaemic shock and active bleeding following a secondary tonsillar haemorrhage. He has a haemoglobin level of 5.5 g/dL on a blood gas. You advise that the boy requires resuscitation including blood transfusion and return to theatre to arrest the haemorrhage. The boy informs you that he is a Jehovah's Witness and he forbids you to perform a blood transfusion. What is the next most appropriate action?**

    A. Call a senior colleague and ask them to come in to give a second opinion
    B. Call the blood bank to find a cell saver device
    C. Perform the blood transfusion as clinically indicated
    D. Contact the hospital lawyer for advice
    E. Perform all measures necessary except the transfusion

13. **A child's trachea is narrowed from its normal diameter of 8 mm to 4 mm. What effect is this likely to have on the airflow during quiet breathing?**

    A. A 4-fold increase in resistance
    B. A 8-fold increase in resistance
    C. A 12-fold increase in resistance
    D. A 16-fold increase in resistance
    E. A 256-fold increase in resistance

14. **What is the most common soft tissue malignancy in childhood?**

    A. Osteosarcoma
    B. Rhabdomyosarcoma
    C. Fibro-ossifying sarcoma
    D. Haemangiopericytoma
    E. Neurofibrosarcoma

15. **Which of the following statements concerning microtia is correct?**

    A. Bilateral microtia is more common than unilateral pathology
    B. The auricle is formed from first branchial arch derivatives
    C. The six hillocks of His form the auricle
    D. The auricle is full-sized at birth
    E. Surgery to repair the atretic ear canal is usually performed at the time of auricular reconstruction

16. **A 4-year-old child presents with a rapidly enlarging right parotid mass and facial palsy. Ultrasonography confirms an intraparotid mass. What is the most common malignant process in this situation?**

    A. Squamous cell carcinoma
    B. Lymphoma
    C. Mucoepidermoid carcinoma
    D. Rhabdomyosarcoma
    E. Adenoid cystic cell carcinoma

17. Concerning Usher syndrome, which of the following statements is false?

A. If both parents are carriers of the defective gene, the chance of having a child with the syndrome is 25%

B. Usher syndrome type 1 is associated with reduced vestibular function

C. Usher syndrome type 2 is less common than type 1

D. Retinitis pigmentosa results in blindness

E. Usher syndrome type 1 is associated with a predominantly low-tone hearing loss

18. Concerning the development of the upper aerodigestive tract, which of the following statements is false?

A. The larynx develops in part from the fourth–sixth branchial arches

B. At birth, the larynx is higher in the neck than in the adult and descends through the first two decades of life

C. The laryngeal musculature develops in part from the fourth branchial arch

D. Laryngomalacia is the commonest cause of infantile stridor

E. Laryngomalacia is commoner in premature infants with neuromuscular immaturity

19. Which of the following statements concerning cutaneous haemangiomas is true?

A. Haemangiomas are considered vascular malformations

B Haemangiomas are always present at birth

C. Surgical removal of a haemangioma is the primary treatment

D. A port wine stain is a cutaneous haemangioma involving the face

E. Subglottic haemangiomas are frequently associated with cutaneous lesions

20. In the Myer–Cotton grading of subglottic stenosis, a 60% stenosis would be:

A. Grade I

B. Grade II

C. Grade III

D. Grade IV

E. None of the above

21. Concerning choanal atresia, which of the following statements is true?

A. It may be associated with genital defects

B. Is always apparent at birth

C. Is usually not apparent until teenage years

D. Is usually bilateral

E. Is more common in males

22. **Regarding tracheo-oesophageal fistula, which of the following statements is true?**
    A. It is more common in females
    B. Type II is the most common type
    C. It has an association with dystopia canthorum
    D. It has a close association with vascular anomalies
    E. It may be diagnosed on antenatal ultrasonography

23. **A cutaneous capillary vascular malformation typically:**
    A. Is not obvious at birth, but grows rapidly in the first year of life
    B. Involutes between the ages of 2 and 9 years
    C. Is more common in males
    D. May be associated with underlying meningeal vascular malformations
    E. Does not respond to laser therapy

24. **Which of the following is least associated with Down syndrome?**
    A. Low-set ears
    B. Subglottic stenosis
    C. Subglottic haemangioma
    D. Otitis media with effusion
    E. Relative IgA deficiency

25. **All of the following are associated with Gorlin syndrome except which?**
    A. Meningiomas
    B. Skin basal cell carcinomas
    C. Odontogenic keratocysts
    D. Choanal atresia
    E. Autosomal dominant inheritance

26. **A child is undergoing a rigid bronchoscopy. During the procedure it is noted that the patient's right arm has become pale and pulseless. The arm becomes pink and with a good pulse on removal of the bronchoscope. Compression of which vessel is likely to be the cause of this phenomenon?**
    A. Right common carotid artery
    B. Left common carotid artery
    C. Brachiocephalic artery
    D. Right subclavian vein
    E. Right vertebral artery

27. **Bat ear deformities as a result of a lack of an antihelical fold are due to abnormal development of which structure?**
    A. First hillock of His
    B. Second hillock of His
    C. Third hillock of His
    D. Fourth hillock of His
    E. Fifth hillock of His

28. **You are asked to see a 14-year-old girl with a 3-day history of a painful left neck. On examination she is diffusely tender along the sternocleidomastoid mastoid muscle but there is no focal mass. She has a low-grade fever and a raised C-reactive protein (CRP) (42) but is otherwise well. She is known to suffer from homocystinuria. From the history and examination, what is the most likely diagnosis?**
    A. Acute lymphoblastic leukaemia
    B. Internal jugular vein thrombosis
    C. Rhabdomyosarcoma
    D. Common carotid artery thrombosis
    E. Carotid body tumour

29. **You are referred a 6-year-old boy with a history of a choking episode while playing 2 days ago. His chest X-ray is shown.**

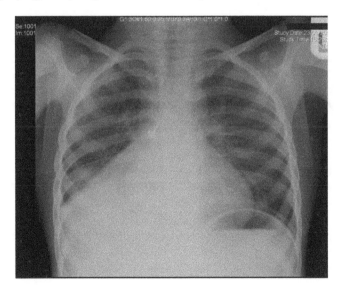

You plan to take him to the operating theatre. What would be the most appropriate method of induction of anaesthesia in this case?

A. Rapid sequence induction and orotracheal intubation
B. Propofol intravenous induction and orotracheal intubation
C. Propofol intravenous induction and laryngeal mask airway placement
D. Gas induction and nasopharyngeal tube insertion
E. Gas induction and orotracheal intubation

30. **You are asked to see a 2-year-old child with suspected sinusitis. Which of the following sinuses is unlikely to be involved?**

A. Sphenoid
B. Ethmoid
C. Maxillary
D. All of the above: a child of this age would not develop sinusitis
E. They all have an equal chance of being involved

31. **What is the most appropriate method of calculating the circulating blood volume of a 2-year-old child?**

A. 5% of body weight
B. 20% of body weight
C. 20 mL/kg
D. 40 mL/kg
E. 80 mL/kg

32. **A mother attends the clinic with her 3-year-old son. She tells you that he has had three episodes of green rhinorrhoea in the last 18 months. Each of these has lasted 2 weeks, between times the child has been well and is healthy on examination. She is concerned about his immune status. What is the most appropriate course of action?**

A. Arrange immunoglobulin testing
B. Schedule the child for examination of the nose under anaesthetic and perform bilateral antral washouts (BAWO)
C. Prescribe a 2-month course of prophylactic low-dose antibiotics
D. Reassure the mother and discharge the child
E. Reassure the mother and review the child in 4 months

33. **Regarding the first branchial arch, which of the following statements is false?**

A. Skeletal components include Meckel's cartilage, the malleus, and the incus
B. The first branchial arch cleft contributes to all three layers of the tympanic membrane
C. Work classified first branchial arch fistulas into type 1 and type 2
D. Type 1 is composed of ectoderm
E. Type 2 is intimately related to the parotid gland and facial nerve

34. **A 5-month-old baby presents with bilateral preauricular sinuses and a discharging pit at the anterior border of sternocleidomastoid. A diagnosis of branchio-oto-renal syndrome (BOR) is suspected. Which of the following statements regarding BOR syndrome is false?**
    A. Hearing loss affects more than 80% of patients with BOR
    B. It affects 1 in 40,000 children
    C. It is an autosomal recessive inherited condition
    D. It may present with conductive or sensorineural hearing loss
    E. It accounts for 2% of profoundly deaf children

35. **Which of the following statements regarding the third and fourth branchial arches is false?**
    A. The only muscle derived from the third arch is the stylopharyngeus
    B. The third branchial arch contributes to the lesser horn and upper body of the hyoid bone
    C. Third and fourth branchial cleft anomalies may present with recurrent thyroiditis
    D. Third branchial cleft fistulas pierce the thyrohyoid membrane and enter the lateral wall of the pyriform fossa
    E. Fistulae may be treated endoscopically initially

36. **Microlaryngoscopy and bronchoscopy (MLB) anaesthesia: which of the following are not generally involved in general anaesthesia for a routine diagnostic paediatric MLB?**
    A. Anticholinergic medications
    B. Local anaesthetic spray
    C. Spontaneous ventilation
    D. Gas induction
    E. Muscle relaxants

37. **A 2-year-old 11 kg boy with a persistent purulent runny nose and clinical suspicion of obstructive sleep apnoea presents to his local district general hospital. A sleep study shows an apnoea–hypopnea index (AHI) of 15. How would you proceed?**
    A. List the child for an adenoidectomy
    B. List the child for an adenotonsillectomy
    C. Refer the child to the nearest tertiary centre performing paediatric ENT
    D. List the child for an adenotonsillectomy and ensure the on-call paediatrician is available that day
    E. Treat with a 2-week course of antibiotics and nasal steroid and review the patient in a few months

38. **You perform an ultrasound scan in a child with persistent cervical lymphadenopathy. Which of the following are high-risk/suspicious features of malignancy in children with lymphadenopathy (more than one apply)?**
    A. Supraclavicular lymph nodes
    B. Lymph nodes larger than 3 cm
    C. Increased hilar blood flow
    D. Ovoid lymph nodes
    E. Skin discoloration

39. **Non-tuberculous mycobacteria (NTB): which of the following statements is false?**
    A. Commonly *Mycobacterium avium–intracellulare* complex in 80% of cases
    B. Usually presents with a warm painless mass and discoloration of the overlying skin
    C. Atypical mycobacteria are acid-fast bacilli which are naturally found in soil and water environments
    D. NTB lymphadenitis commonly presents in children under 5
    E. Common sites for lymphadenitis in order of incidence is submandibular region, preauricular region, and parotid gland

40. **A baby is due to undergo newborn hearing screening programme (NHSP)/congenital hearing loss investigations after spending 72 hours in a neonatal intensive care unit (NICU) when born. Which of the following investigations should be arranged as first line in this child?**
    A. Distraction testing
    B. Automated otoacoustic emission (OAE)
    C. Automated OAE and full audiological assessment at 6 months
    D. Automated OAE and auditory brainstem response (ABR)
    E. ABR and a MRI scan

41. **Imaging when investigating paediatric hearing loss may show a number of abnormalities. Which of the following statements is false?**
    A. Usher syndrome is associated with semicircular canal aplasia
    B. A Mondini dysplasia is the combination of an abnormal apical cochlear with an enlarged vestibular aqueduct
    C. Radiological findings of X-linked deafness included a widened internal auditory meatus and enlarged vestibular aqueduct
    D. MRI scans are useful for imaging the contents of the internal auditory canal
    E. Radiology may be normal when hearing loss is associated with a viral infective aetiology

42. **You perform microlaryngoscopy and bronchoscopy (MLB) on a 6-month-old child with increasing inspiratory stridor and see subglottic haemangioma obstructing 40% of the airway. The child is not desaturating and is able to feed although hasn't been gaining weight appropriately. What would be the appropriate management?**
    A. Endoscopic debridement of the haemangioma
    B. Intralesional steroid injections followed by a trial of propranolol
    C. Endoscopic laser treatment followed by a trial of propranolol
    D. A trial of propranolol commenced as an inpatient with serial MLB follow-up
    E. Open airway surgery to remove the haemangioma

43. **Concerning paediatric tracheostomy, which of the following statements is false?**
    A. Non-dissolvable stay sutures may be inserted until the first tracheostomy tube change
    B. Maturation sutures involve the placement of sutures between the stomal skin and the anterior tracheal wall
    C. A vertical tracheotomy is commonly performed
    D. Surgical tracheostomy should be followed by a postoperative chest X-ray
    E. Removing a plug of subcutaneous fat is usually not required in neonates

44. **Craniosynostosis and associated syndromes: which of the following statements is false?**
    A. Ossification of the cranial vault starts at the centre of each cranial bone and extends outwards towards the suture lines
    B. Brachycephaly refers to early bicoronal suture fusion
    C. Secondary craniosynostosis refers to early suture fusion due to primary failure of brain growth
    D. Children with Crouzon syndrome may have cognitive disabilities
    E. Children with Apert syndrome may have cognitive disabilities and syndactyly of their hands and feet

45. **An 11-month-old child presents with an enlarging mass over the dorsum of the nose that has a negative Furstenberg's sign. Which of the following is the most likely diagnosis?**
    A. Encephalocoele
    B. Meningocoele
    C. Nasolabial cyst
    D. Dermoid cyst
    E. Thornwald't cyst

46. Regarding cytomegalovirus infection, which of the following statements is false?

A. Congenital hearing loss due to congenital cytomegalovirus infection is usually present by the age of 2 years

B. 90% of babies born with congenital cytomegalovirus are asymptomatic

C. Cytomegalovirus testing is performed using blood from the Guthrie card

D. Ganciclovir is used in the treatment of symptomatic babies

E. Cytomegalovirus is one of the human herpesviruses otherwise known as HHV-5

47. A child with a confirmed *RET* mutation who has a family history of multiple endocrine neoplasia should undergo:

A. Serial neck ultrasound scan for lifelong surveillance

B. Serial thyroid ultrasound scans and if normal for 5 years can be discharged

C. Prophylactic hemithyroidectomy

D. Prophylactic total thyroidectomy

E. Total thyroidectomy with central neck dissection

48. Congenital laryngeal webs: which of the following statements is false?

A. Congenital laryngeal webs are associated with chromosome 22q11.2 microdeletion syndrome in 50% of cases

B. Cardiac abnormalities are seen in 50% of patients with chromosome 22q11.2 syndrome

C. In the prenatal period, laryngeal atresia may be seen on an ultrasound scan as features of CHAOS (congenital high airway obstructive syndrome)

D. Congenital laryngeal webs result from degrees of failure of the epithelium's resorption during the 17th and 20th weeks of intrauterine development

E. A congenital web may present with stridor

49. A 4-year-old otherwise well child presents to clinic with persistent drooling, sometimes having to change their top during the day as it is soaked. The child has large tonsils and symptoms of obstructive sleep apnoea. What is the most appropriate initial management of this child?

A. Consider Botox injections to the submandibular gland

B. Discuss submandibular rerouting if no significant change by age 6

C. Discuss performing an adenotonsillectomy as the child has sleep apnoea

D. Prescribed anticholinergic medications such as hyoscine patches

E. Behavioural modification in conjunction with an assessment by speech and language therapy

50. **A 2-year-old has been referred for an ENT assessment as they have had six episodes of croup. Which statement regarding the croup is false?**

A. Croup is usually viral caused by the parainfluenza virus (a paramyxovirus)

B. Common bacterial pathogens causing croup include *Staphylococcus aureus, Streptococcus pneumoniae,* and *Haemophilus influenza*

C. Steeple sign refers to subglottic changes seen on a chest X-ray in croup

D. Patients with recurrent croup should be investigated for tracheomalacia

E. The cricoid is located at C4 at birth and C6 in an adult

51. **A 4-month-old baby has been referred for an airway assessment. They were born at 32 weeks, were intubated for a week, and went on to have surgery to ligate a patent ductus arteriosus (PDA). They now have a soft stridor worse on exertion and a hoarse voice. Which of these is the least likely pathology to be encountered during microlaryngoscopy and bronchoscopy?**

A. Subglottic stenosis

B. Subglottic cysts

C. Vocal cord palsy

D. Tracheomalacia

E. Laryngeal web

52. **The national tracheostomy safety project led to the design of laminated posters above the bed of all patients with a tracheostomy. When performing a new tracheostomy in a child, which of the following information is required on these posters?**

A. Size of suction catheter to be used

B. Depth of suction in centimetres

C. Number and place of any sutures left

D. Grade of laryngoscopy

E. All of the above

1. E. This is a first branchial cleft fistula (collaural fistula). These congenital fistulas can take a course close to the facial nerve. From the possible answers given, MRI is the most appropriate answer, although some surgeons would proceed to surgery directly, with identification of the facial nerve via a modified Blair ('lazy S') incision.

2. B. The Eustachian tube is normally closed. It is opened by contraction of the tensor veli palatini muscle.

3. E. Cyanotic episodes and failure to thrive suggest severe laryngomalacia. In these instances, further intervention is indicated.

4. B. This is likely to be a haematoma of the sternocleidomastoid muscle. Conservative and supportive measures are the most appropriate first stage of therapy.

5. C. The father has the legal responsibility for the child and can consent to the procedure.

Consent need only be given by one person with parental responsibility but it is good practice to involve both parents.

The law in relation to parental responsibility has been revised. Originally those people with parental responsibility were described in the Children Act 1989. They included both the child's parents if they were married at the time of conception or birth or the child's mother if they were not married. Fathers not married to the mother could have acquired parental responsibility through a court order, subsequent agreement, or marriage.

However, more recently the law has been changed to recognize unmarried fathers and so in relation to children born after 1 December 2003 (England and Wales), 15 April 2002 (Northern Ireland), or 4 May 2006 (Scotland), both of a child's legal parents have parental responsibility if they are registered on the child's birth certificate. This applies irrespective of whether the parents are married or not.

6. D. The inner ear develops first as the otic placode forms in week 3 of gestation and the semicircular canals are fully formed by week 8.

The ossicles are adult-sized at birth. The auricle develops from condensations of mesoderm of the first and second branchial arches. These give rise to the six hillocks of His. At birth, the auricle is adult-shaped but is not adult-sized until approximately 9 years.

The bony labyrinth develops from 14 centres of ossification.

7. C. Auricular formation occurs in the first trimester. By week 12 the auricle is formed by fusion of the hillocks of His and is adult-shaped by week 20. Formation of the middle ear begins at week

10 and the ossicles are adult-sized by 16 weeks. The external ear canal develops from the ectoderm of first pharyngeal groove. This forms a solid core which does not hollow out until week 28.

8. B. This child is in type I shock (up to 15% blood volume loss). The circulating volume of a child is approximately 80 mL/kg. Therefore the child has lost up to 120 mL of blood.

9. C. HPV subtypes 6 and 11 are associated with recurrent respiratory papillomatosis and are also associated with genital warts. HPV types 16 and 18 have most often been associated with cancer in the genital area.

10. E. Gardasil HPV vaccine protects against HPV strains 6, 11, 16, and 18.

11. E. Pendred syndrome is the most common syndromal form of deafness and is associated with developmental abnormalities of the cochlea, sensorineural hearing loss, and goitre.

Pendred syndrome is associated with temporal bone abnormalities ranging from a large vestibular aqueduct to the Mondini malformation. It is inherited in an autosomal recessive pattern of inheritance so that the chance of a subsequent child with the condition is one in four.

The condition is caused by a defect in the organification of iodine. The perchlorate test is used in the diagnosis of Pendred syndrome. The test is performed by administering radiolabelled iodine and measuring the radioactivity emitted from the thyroid. Potassium perchlorate is then administered. This is a competitive inhibitor of iodide transport into the thyroid. The emittance of radioactivity is again measured over the thyroid and compared to the initial result.

In unaffected individuals, the amount of radiolabelled iodine in the thyroid remains stable due to the rapid oxidation of iodide to iodine and its subsequent incorporation into thyroglobulin.

In affected individuals, the transport of iodine is delayed, resulting in iodide passing into the blood. This manifests as a decrease in radiolabelled iodine in the thyroid.

12. C. An adult Jehovah's Witness can refuse a blood transfusion. However, a minor cannot refuse a transfusion if it is required for a life-saving procedure, even if deemed competent.

13. D. This relates to Poiseuille's law, which states that resistance to airflow is inversely proportional to the fourth power of the airway radius when laminar flow is present. Therefore, if the radius is halved, without altering the length or viscosity, then the resistance increases 16-fold.

14. B. Rhabdomyosarcoma is the most common soft tissue malignancy in childhood and occurs most commonly in the head and neck.

15. C. The majority of cases of microtia are unilateral (90%). The auricle is formed from the six hillocks of His, three from each of the first and second branchial arches, and at birth the auricle is approximately 65% of adult size.

Surgery to the atretic ear canal is controversial and in a unilateral microtia with contralateral normal hearing is not usually undertaken due to the poor results, as middle ear abnormalities are associated with microtia.

16. C. Mucoepidermoid carcinoma is the commonest malignant salivary gland tumour in children. Most are low grade and have a good prognosis.

17. E. Usher syndrome is inherited in an autosomal recessive pattern. Type 1 is the commonest and is associated with profound congenital deafness, abnormal vestibular function, and retinitis pigmentosa occurring in the first decade of life.

Type 2 is associated with a moderate to severe congenital deafness, normal vestibular function, and retinitis pigmentosa occurring in the second or third decade of life.

18. E. The exact aetiology of laryngomalacia is unknown but it is not commoner in premature infants.

19. E. Up to 50% of patients with a subglottic haemangioma will have a cutaneous lesion. However, of those patients with a cutaneous lesion only a small percentage will have a subglottic haemangioma.

Haemangiomas are benign vascular tumours that appear after birth, while vascular malformations are present at birth. In general, surgery is reserved for those tumours not responding to either conservative treatment with observation, steroids, or laser ablation, or which are in a position to cause problems such as to the eye.

A port wine stain is a cutaneous capillary vascular malformation.

20. B. The Myer–Cotton grading system describes the percentage of tracheal stenosis:

- Grade I: 0–50%
- Grade II: 51–70%
- Grade III: 71–99%
- Grade IV: complete obstruction.

Stridor at rest occurs in stenoses of approximately grade III and above.

21. A. Choanal atresia may be seen as part of the CHARGE (Colomba, Heart defects, Atresia choanae, Retarded growth, Genital defects, Ear anomalies) syndrome, or with Treacher Collins syndrome. Unilateral atresia which is most common may not present until later in childhood. It is more common in females.

22. E. Tracheo-oesophageal fistulas are more common in males and type I is the most common. There is rarely an association with vascular anomalies. Impairment of fetal swallowing may lead to polyhydramnios on ultrasonography.

Dystopia canthorum is associated with Waardenburg syndrome.

23. D. Vascular malformations are typically visible at birth, but may be difficult to find and whereas cutaneous haemangiomas involute between 2 and 9 years of age, vascular malformations do not. There is an equal incidence in males and females.

The Surge–Weber syndrome consists of a cutaneous capillary vascular malformation and an underlying intracranial vascular malformation.

Cutaneous capillary vascular malformations typically do respond to laser therapy, particularly pulsed dye lasers and argon lasers.

24. C. Down syndrome is associated with an increased risk of all of the listed options except subglottic haemangioma. The relative IgA deficiency predisposes these children to upper respiratory tract infections.

25. D. Gorlin syndrome (Gorlin–Goliz syndrome) is associated with:

- multiple basal cell carcinomas
- cutaneous abnormalities
- skeletal anomalies
- cranial calcifications
- multiple odontogenic keratocysts.

26. C. The right arm is supplied with blood by the right subclavian artery, a branch of the brachiocephalic artery, which often passes obliquely across the trachea and may become compressed during bronchoscopy.

27. D. The auricle develops from the six hillocks of His. The first three from the first branchial arch and the latter three from the second. The first three hillocks form the tragus, helical crus, and helix. The fourth hillock forms the antihelix, the fifth the scapha, and the sixth the lobule.

28. B. Homocystinuria is an inherited autosomal recessive disorder of methionine metabolism. This causes a widespread disorder of the connective tissue, muscles, central nervous system, and cardiovascular system, often with a marfanoid appearance.

Thrombotic complications are common, affecting the venous and arterial vasculature. These complications often result in death before the age of 30. From the clinical scenario described, it is likely that the child would be more unwell if thrombosis of the common carotid artery had occurred.

29. D. This child requires rigid bronchoscopy to retrieve the pin in the right main bronchus. This is best achieved by performing a gas induction and placing a nasopharyngeal tube, allowing the child to breathe spontaneously while the procedure is performed.

30. A. The development of the sinuses proceeds as follows:

- Maxillary sinuses are present at birth.
- Ethmoid sinuses are present at birth.
- Sphenoid sinus pneumatization starts in the third year of life.
- Frontal sinuses are not present at birth and are not aerated before 6 years of age.

31. E. The circulating volume of a child is 8–9% of body weight, or 80 mL/kg. The hourly fluid maintenance for a child is:

- 4 mL/kg for the first 10 kg
- then add 2 mL/kg for the next 10 kg
- then add 1 mL/kg for any weight after 20 kg.

Example: a 25 kg child requires:

- 4 mL × 10 kg = 40
- Plus 2 mL × 10 kg = 20
- Plus 1 mL × 5 kg = 5
- Total: 40 + 20 + 5 = 65 mL/hour

A child in shock should receive a fluid challenge of 20 mL/kg of crystalloid. A further two fluid challenge boluses of 20 mL/kg may be given if the child does not respond.

32. D. It is not unusual for a healthy child to have at least three upper respiratory tract infections per year. No specific investigations are required and the mother should be reassured.

33. B. The first branchial arch cartilage is otherwise known as Meckel's cartilage which forms the incus, malleus, sphenomandibular ligament, and the lingula of the mandible. The tympanic membrane is formed of three layers. The superficial ectodermal layer and the middle mesodermal layer are formed from the first branchial cleft. The first branchial pouch contributes to the mucosal layer (endoderm) of the tympanic membrane, the middle ear, and Eustachian tube. Abnormalities of the first branchial cleft are commonly classified by the Work classification system, but other classification systems have been described by Arnot and Olsen

34. C. Branchio-oto-renal syndrome is an autosomal dominant inherited condition involving mutations of the *EYA1, SIX1,* and *SIX5* genes. Hearing loss may be mixed, conductive, or sensorineural and a variety of temporal bone abnormalities have been seen on CT scans of these patients. Abnormalities of the second branchial arch such as cyst sinuses and fistulas are extremely common.

35. B. Third and fourth branchial arch abnormalities are rare and often present as recurrent deep space neck infections or thyroiditis. The third branchial arch contributes to the greater horn and lower body of the hyoid bone while the fourth brachial arch contributes to the laryngeal cartilages.

36. E. Where possible, a diagnostic MLB in the paediatric population is performed under anaesthesia whereby the patient is spontaneously ventilating. This is best achieved using inhaled agents such as sevoflurane, often delivered through a nasopharyngeal airway. Anticholinergic may be administered to reduce secretions and a local anaesthetic spray to the larynx enables instrumentation without laryngospasm.

37. C. This child has severe obstructive sleep apnoea as defined by an obstructive AHI of >10. This combined with the clinical symptoms of a persistent purulent nasal discharge make them a candidate for an adenotonsillectomy. As per British Association of Paediatric Otolaryngology guidance, children with severe obstructive sleep apnoea under 15 kg are unsuitable for adenotonsillectomy in a district general hospital setting and should therefore be referred to a tertiary centre.

38. A, B, C. Malignant lymph nodes are large, round, with an absent hilum. They are hypoechoic with irregular and invasive borders. Structural changes such as intranodal necrosis and calcification may be present and in general an increase in hilar blood flow.

39. B. NTB often presents in young children aged under 5 with a cold painless firm mass. The mass may enlarge, become fluctuant, and discolour the skin to form the classical 'violaceous hue'.

40. D. The NHSP consists of two pathways: the well baby pathway and the special care baby unit (SCBU/NICU) baby pathway. Babies who have spent 48 hours in SCBU or NICU should be referred through the second pathway where the first-line screening investigations consist of both an automated OAE and an automated ABR.

41. A. CHARGE syndrome is associated with semicircular canal aplasia.

42. D. The use of propranolol is now recognized as a safe and efficacious treatment for infantile haemangioma of the airway. In such cases, propranolol should only be commenced as an inpatient after a full cardiovascular and respiratory review. The treatment is started at a dose of 1 mg/kg/day in three divided doses and increased to 2 mg/kg/day after 1 week of therapy. The blood pressure and heart rate should be monitored very carefully throughout the treatment. Serial endoscopic follow-up should be arranged to monitor the effect of treatment.

43. E. Performing paediatric tracheostomy requires careful positioning of the patient. This is often best achieved with a head ring and shoulder bag/bolster and strapping of the neck to tighten the skin and subcutaneous tissue over the trachea. Removing a large plug of subcutaneous fat allows a much better view of the strap muscles and trachea. Maturation sutures raise the anterior tracheal wall to the skin to create a stable stoma which is easy to cannulate in the event of an accidental decannulation.

44. D. Craniosynostosis refers to the premature fusion of one or more cranial sutures due to a primary defect of ossification (primary craniosynostosis) or a failure of brain growth (secondary craniosynostosis). Fibroblast growth factor receptor (FGFR)-related craniosynostosis refers to a number of syndromes with defects in the *FGFR* gene. Patients with Crouzon syndrome have a mutation of the *FGFR2* gene and have normal intelligence.

45. D. A dermoid cyst is derived from ectoderm and mesoderm and presents as a slow-growing painless mass anywhere from the glabella of the nose to the tip. About 20% may show an intracranial communication, hence a preoperative MRI scan is mandatory.

46. A. Hearing loss associated with cytomegalovirus infection is usually progressive.

47. D. Patients with multiple endocrine neoplasia 2 (MEN2) have mutations of the *RET* proto-oncogene and are at significant risk of medullary thyroid cancer. In MEN2B/3, medullary thyroid cancer is aggressive and may manifest as metastatic disease in infancy, hence prophylactic total thyroidectomy in those with confirmed mutations is recommended within the first year of life. Those with MEN2A are advised to undergo prophylactic total thyroidectomy by the age of 5 years.

48. D. Congenital laryngeal webs result from degrees of failure of the epithelium's resorption during the 8th to 10th weeks of intrauterine development. Cohen classified these as types as I–IV depending on the degree of glottic narrowing (type I, 0–35%; type 2, 35–55%; type 3, 55–75%; type 4, >75%).

49. E. In an otherwise normal child, the initial management of drooling should be conservative. History and examination should include information on feeding history, dental hygiene, nasal obstruction, and general neuromuscular development. In a non-neurological child, every effort should be made to encourage oral control in conjunction with oromotor exercises and behavioural modifications. Optimizing the nasal and oral airway is advisable.

50. D. Children who present with recurrent croup should have a full ENT assessment and be investigated for subglottic stenosis. An MLB should be undertaken and the airway sized.

51. E. Neonates who have been intubated at birth are at risk of multiple airway defects. Most commonly prolonged intubation can lead to subglottic cysts followed by an acquired subglottic stenosis. Traumatic intubation can cause cricoarytenoid joint dislocation and therefore vocal cord palsy. Left recurrent laryngeal nerve is also at risk during a PDA ligation.

52. E. The national tracheostomy safety project led to the design of a laminated poster above the head of every patient with a tracheostomy.

1. **A 42-year-old male presents with nasal obstruction. A computed tomography (CT) scan of the paranasal sinuses is reported as showing opacification of the right maxillary sinus with 'double density' signals throughout the sinus. Which of the following is the least likely pathology?**
    A. Allergic fungal sinusitis
    B. Chondrosarcoma
    C. Inverted papilloma
    D. Antrochoanal polyp
    E. Ossifying fibroma

2. **Concerning nasal ciliary physiology and anatomy, which of the following statements is least accurate?**
    A. The nose is lined by ciliated pseudostratified glandular columnar epithelium
    B. The nasal cilia are arranged as nine microtubule doublets formed in an outer circle around a central pair
    C The outer microtubular doublets are linked by the protein nexin
    D. Ciliary movement is described as having two phases
    E. Normal ciliary beat frequency is approximately 10–25 beats per minute

3. **Which of the following bones is least likely to be transected as part of an endoscopic transethmoidal sphenoidotomy?**
    A. Uncinate process
    B. Bulla ethmoidalis
    C. Anterior wall of the sphenoid
    D. Palatine bone
    E. Ground lamella of the middle turbinate

4. **When performing an external ethmoidectomy, at what distance from the anterior lacrimal crest are you most likely to find the posterior ethmoidal artery?**

    A. 12 mm
    B. 24 mm
    C. 30 mm
    D. 36 mm
    E. 42 mm

5. **Which of the following bones do not form part of the osteology of the lateral nasal wall?**

    A. Maxilla
    B. Palatine
    C. Ethmoid
    D. Perpendicular plate of the sphenoid
    E. Inferior turbinate

6. **In a 70 kg male being prepared for a lymph node biopsy under local anaesthetic, what is the maximum volume of 2% lidocaine without adrenaline that can be injected?**

    A. 5 ml
    B. 10 ml
    C 15 ml
    D 20 ml
    E. 25 ml

7. **Ohngren's line is used as a prognostic indicator in management of carcinoma of the maxillary sinus. This line is described as an imaginary plane perpendicular to the intersection between:**

    A. The lateral canthus and the angle of the jaw
    B. The lateral canthus and the menton
    C. The medial canthus and the angle of the jaw
    D. The tragus and the nasal tip
    E. The tragus and the menton

8. **While performing functional endoscopic sinus (FES) surgery, you are operating to remove the anterior ethmoidal air cells when you see clear fluid flowing from the region of the lateral lamella of the cribriform plate. What is the next most appropriate action?**

    A. Stop surgery, wake the patient up, and see if the clear fluid continues
    B. Inject intrathecal fluorescein to confirm the presence of a cerebrospinal fluid (CSF) leak
    C. Perform a local repair of the probable CSF leak
    D. Continue the surgery, then pack the nose with a nasal tampon for 48 hours
    E. Request the neurosurgeons to perform a craniotomy and dural repair

9. **A 14-year-old boy presents with a unilateral nasal mass. A coronal short TI inversion recovery (STIR) image from the magnetic resonance imaging (MRI) is shown. The lesion fills the nasal cavity and involves the pterygopalatine fossa. What is the most appropriate management plan?**

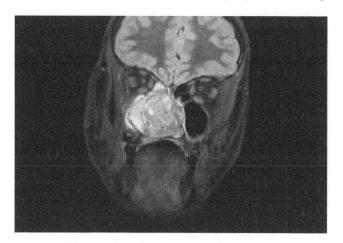

   A. Observe with serial MRI scans
   B. Arrange external beam radiotherapy
   C. Perform a biopsy to confirm the diagnosis
   D. Arrange for surgery to be performed
   E. Arrange arterial embolization

10. **A 46-year-old man presents with a exophytic tumour arising from his right maxillary antrum extending onto the hard palate and anterior maxillary wall only. It has not invaded the orbital walls or involved his subcutaneous tissues. A biopsy is reported as squamous cell carcinoma. According to the TNM (8th edition) classification, what stage would this tumour be?**
   A. T1
   B. T2
   C. T3
   D. T4a
   E. T4b

11. **You wish to use a urinary catheter as a postnasal pack in a patient with epistaxis. The only available size is a French size 24. What is the diameter of the tube?**
   A. 4 mm
   B. 6 mm
   C. 8 mm
   D. 10 mm
   E. 12 mm

12. **Which of the following does not form part of the bony orbital cavity?**

 A. Lacrimal bone
 B. Zygomatic bone
 C. Palatine bone
 D. Greater wing of the sphenoid
 E. Nasal bone

13. **A patient presents with cerebrospinal fluid (CSF) rhinorrhoea. What are the likely signal characteristics of CSF on MRI?**

 A. High-intensity signal on T1-weighted imaging
 B. Low-intensity signal on T2-weighted imaging
 C. High-intensity signal on T2-weighted imaging
 D. Enhancement following administration of gadolinium
 E. MRI poorly identifies CSF

14. **Which of the following statements best describes granulomatosis with polyangiitis (GPA; formerly known as Wegner's granulomatosis)?**

 A. Untreated, the disease is usually asymptomatic for many years
 B. Cirrhosis of the liver is a common feature of the disease
 C. The perinuclear antineutrophil cytoplasmic antibody (pANCA) is highly sensitive for the disease
 D. It is most common in those of Afro-Caribbean origin
 E. The cytoplasmic antineutrophil cytoplasmic antibody (cANCA) is highly sensitive for the disease

15. **A 44-year-male with a 4-month history of anosmia reports that he can still smell ammonia. Which cranial nerve is likely to be responsible for this?**

 A. One—olfactory
 B. Five—trigeminal
 C. Seven—facial
 D. Nine—glossopharyngeal
 E. Ten—vagus

16. **Concerning the embryology of the nose and paranasal sinuses, which of the following statements is false?**

 A. The frontal sinus originates from pneumatization of the frontal recess and is usually not visible at birth
 B. At 2 years of age, the floor of the maxillary sinus is usually higher than the floor of the nasal cavity
 C. Failure of resorption of the nasobuccal membrane results in choanal atresia
 D. An absence of nasal bones on intrauterine screening is associated with Down syndrome
 E. Branchio-oto-renal syndrome is characterized by abnormal cilia function and chronic sinusitis

17. According to the Lund–Mackay grading system for sinus opacification, what would be the score for this CT scan of the paranasal sinuses?

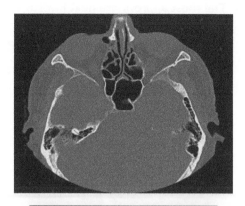

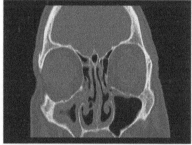

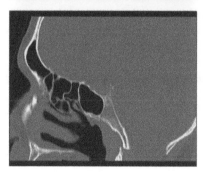

A. Zero
B. Two
C. Six
D. Eight
E. Ten

18. **A 60-year-old man is referred by his general practitioner (GP) with unilateral nasal obstruction. The GP has organized for him to have a CT scan before the appointment. The most appropriate next investigation would be:**

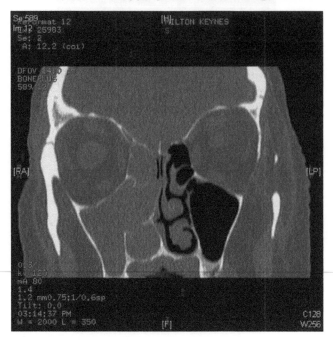

A. Referral to the head and neck multidisciplinary team
B. Referral to the specialist rhinologist in your hospital
C. Schedule the patient for endoscopic sinus surgery
D. Schedule the patient for biopsy
E. Arrange an MRI of the neck to examine nodal status

19. **Which of the following is not closely related to the frontal recess?**

A. Agger nasi
B. Ethmoidal bulla
C. Middle turbinate
D. Lamina papyracea
E. Superior turbinate

20. **A 79-year-old man presents to the clinic with left-sided nasal discharge and obstruction. A mass is found arising from the ethmoid sinuses and histology shows an adenocarcinoma. Which of the following is the most significant risk factor for developing this disease?**

A. Smoking
B. Alcohol
C. A and B
D. Wood dust
E. Asbestos

21. **Which of the following is least likely to improve the symptoms from an anterior nasal septal perforation?**
    A. Nasal hygiene
    B. Free tissue transfer cartilage graft repair (cartilage, perichondrium only)
    C. Silastic button placement
    D. Local flap repair
    E. Free tissue transfer composite graft repair (epithelium, cartilage, epithelium)

22. **A 4-year-old child has sustained a clean facial laceration which requires closure. Which of the following is the most acceptable form of closure?**
    A. 5/0 silk
    B. 2/0 undyed Vicryl
    C. 4/0 Monocryl
    D. Skin clips
    E. 4/0 dyed Vicryl subcuticular

23. **Concerning rhinoplasty techniques, which of the following techniques is unlikely to achieve the stated aim?**
    A. An onlay graft overlying the alar domes will increase tip projection
    B. Separating the medial crura of the lower lateral cartilages from the septum will decrease tip projection
    C. Removing part of the cranial edge of the lower lateral cartilage 'cephalic shave' will cause caudal tip rotation
    D. Using the lateral crura of the lower lateral cartilages to elongate the medial crura 'lateral crural steel' will increase tip projection
    E. Interdomal sutures will increase tip projection

24. **Concerning facial aesthetic analysis, which of the following statements is false?**
    A. The width of the eye is approximately one-fifth the width of the face
    B. The nasolabial angle describes the nasal projection in relation to the upper lip
    C. The nasolabial angle is more obtuse in Caucasian women than men
    D. A tip projection ratio of 0.6 is ideal (tip projection ratio: radix–tip distance/tip to alar–cheek junction distance)
    E. The hair line to alar base distance represents approximately two-thirds of the facial height

25. **Concerning melanoma, which of the following statements is least likely to be true?**
    A. Tumour thickness and ulceration are the most important histological markers of prognosis
    B. Superficial spreading melanoma has an initial radial growth phase followed by a vertical growth phase
    C. Nodular melanomas are less aggressive than other forms of melanoma
    D. Xeroderma pigmentosa represents an inherited risk of developing melanoma
    E. Fitzpatrick type I skin carries a higher risk of developing melanoma than type VI skin

26. **Which of the following is not used in the American Joint Committee on Cancer (AJCC) staging system for melanoma?**
    A. Tumour thickness
    B. Tumour ulceration
    C. Size of lymph nodes
    D. Number of lymph nodes
    E. Sentinel node biopsy results

27. **The nose is subdivided into how many aesthetic subunits?**
    A. Five
    B. Seven
    C. Eight
    D. Nine
    E. Eleven

28. **A patient suffers a knife wound to the face. The wound is closed primarily, tension free, and forms a well-healed scar. The patient wishes to know how strong the tissue is compared to normal skin. Which answer is most appropriate?**
    A. Compared to normal skin, the tissue is 10% as strong
    B. Compared to normal skin, the tissue is 30% as strong
    C. Compared to normal skin, the tissue is 50% as strong
    D. Compared to normal skin, the tissue is 80% as strong
    E. Compared to normal skin, the tissue is 100% as strong

29. **Which of the following represent the lowest risk of developing a basal cell carcinoma?**
    A. Basal cell nevus syndrome (Gorlin syndrome)
    B. Sun exposure
    C. Xeroderma pigmentosa
    D. Immunosuppression
    E. Fitzpatrick skin type V

30. **A Z-plasty is used on a patient. The advantages include all of the following except:**
    A. Excision of the scar
    B. Shortening of the scar
    C. Lengthening of the scar
    D. Reorientation of the scar
    E. Release tension on the scar

31. **The sural nerve can be used as an interposition cable graft in facial nerve repair. Which of the following statements is false?**
    A. The nerve is found approximately 1 cm posterior to the lateral malleolus
    B. Sectioning the nerve will result in paraesthesia along the lateral aspect of the foot
    C. The nerve contains mixed sensory and motor innervation to the flexor digiti minimi brevis
    D. Up to 40 cm of the nerve can be harvested
    E. It is in close approximation to the short saphenous vein

32. **In normal wound healing, when would you expect the number of fibroblasts to peak?**
    A. Within 6 hours
    B. Within 24 hours
    C. Within 3 days
    D. Between 3 and 5 days
    E. Between 6 and 7 days

33. **The following diagram represents a rhomboid rotational flap. Which of the following statements is correct?**

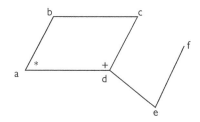

    A. When closing a rhomboid flap, point d is transposed to point a
    B. Angle * is 80 degrees
    C. Angle + is 150 degrees
    D. Up to four separate flaps could be raised
    E. The distance from point c to point f should be as small as possible when using this flap on the face.

34. **Tumours of the lower lip are typically:**
    A. Basal cell carcinomas
    B. Associated with poor oral hygiene
    C. Associated with neck metastases in 45% of patients at presentation
    D. Almost universally in males
    E. Associated with late metastasis in 50%

35. **Which of the following would be the least appropriate recipient site for a full-thickness skin graft?**

A. Pericranium

B. Muscle

C. Fat

D. Cartilage

E. Bone

36. **Which of the following flaps relies on the principle of delayed division of the pedicle?**

A. Dufourmentel flap

B. Abbe flap

C. Karapandzic flap

D. Gillies fan flap

E. Radial forearm flap

37. **Concerning reconstructive flaps, which of the following statements is incorrectly matched?**

A. Latissimus dorsi flap is based on the thoracodorsal artery

B. Pectoralis major flap is based on the thoracoacromial artery

C. Sternocleidomastoid flap is based on the ascending pharyngeal artery

D. Deltopectoral flap is based on the perforating branches of the internal thoracic artery

E. Midline forehead flap is based on the supratrochlear artery

38. **Following excision of a 4 mm diameter basal cell carcinoma from the tip of the nose with a 3 mm margin, which of the following statements describes the least appropriate method of repair?**

A. The use of a full-thickness skin graft, 'Wolfe graft', using postauricular skin

B. The use of a nasolabial advancement flap based on the facial artery

C. Primary closure

D. The use of a paramedian rotational forehead flap based on the supratrochlear artery

E. The use of a bilobed rotation flap

39. **A 65-year-old man presents with a basal cell carcinoma of the lower lip. You decide to resect the lesion and reconstruct using an Abbe flap. Which of the following statements regarding the flap is incorrect?**

A. The Abbe flap is generally used when the lip defect involves one-third to two-thirds of the lip

B. The Abbe flap is generally not used when the defect involves the commissure

C. The Abbe flap can be based on the superior or inferior labial artery

D. The labial artery is a branch of the facial artery and lies deep to the orbicularis oculi muscle

E. The Abbe flap is a single-stage procedure

40. **Concerning reconstructive flaps, which of the following statements can be considered incorrect?**
    A. A full-thickness skin graft contains the epidermis and the whole of the dermis
    B. A full-thickness skin graft will usually give a better cosmetic result than a split skin graft
    C. Most local skin flaps on the face are random pattern flaps deriving their blood supply from the dermal–subdermal plexus
    D. With a local advancement flap, Burrows triangles may allow the flap to sit better
    E. A ratio of 1:2 pedicle width to flap length should be strictly adhered to on the face

41. **The diagram shows the planning for a bilobed (Zitelli) flap to be used on the dorsum of the nose. Which of the following statements is false?**

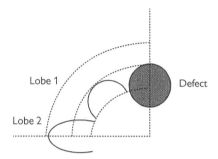

    A. The maximal angle of rotation is 90–100 degrees
    B. The width of lobe 1 should be the same width as the defect
    C. When using this to reconstruct defects on the nose, there is a random pattern blood supply
    D. The most tension when closing is usually found in the defect site
    E A disadvantage of the flap is a complex scar

42. **In which of the following situations would Moh's micrographic surgery be least appropriate?**
    A. A large squamous cell carcinoma on the cheek
    B. A recurrent squamous cell carcinoma on the forehead
    C. Age greater than 80 years
    D. Cosmetically sensitive area
    E. A basal cell carcinoma arising in the posterior triangle of the neck

43. **A 75-year-old man is undergoing a local anaesthetic excision of a suspected basal cell carcinoma on his cheek. What clinical margin of excision is most appropriate?**
    A. 0 mm
    B. 2 mm
    C. 5 mm
    D. 1 cm
    E. 2–3 cm

44. **In relation to the allergic response, which of the following statements is true?**
    A. The early phase of the allergic response is primarily histamine mediated
    B. The early phase of the immune response involves the degranulation of dendritic cells
    C. The early phase occurs within 30–60 minutes of exposure to a previously sensitized antigen
    D. Corticosteroids primarily affect the early phase of the allergic reaction
    E. It never results in cobble-stoning of the posterior pharyngeal wall

45. **Concerning obstructive sleep apnoea (OSA), which of the following statements is false?**
    A. Can lead to hypertension, arrhythmias, and pulmonary hypertension if untreated
    B. As part of the initial investigations the haemoglobin and thyroid function tests should be checked
    C. Collapse of the upper airways is related to the Bernoulli principle
    D. Sleep nasoendoscopy is good at visualizing the level of obstruction, thus assessing benefits of any planned procedure
    E. Obesity hypoventilation syndrome purely depends on the body mass index of the patient

46. **Regarding nasopharyngeal carcinoma, which of the following statements is true?**
    A. The most common site is the midline nasopharynx
    B. It is generally associated with the Epstein–Barr virus
    C. If extension to the parapharyngeal space without paranasal sinus involvement is present, this constitutes a T3 tumour
    D. Surgery is the mainstay of treatment for this disease
    E. Grommets are commonly used for associated middle ear effusion

47. **Concerning tumours of the sinonasal region, which of the following statements is false?**
    A. The most common malignant tumours of the maxillary sinus are epithelial cell in origin
    B. Inverted papilloma is associated with a 10% risk of malignant transformation
    C. The commonest sites of malignant tumours within the nose and paranasal sinuses are the lateral wall, ethmoids, and maxillary sinus
    D. Mucosal melanoma of the nasal cavity which invades the mucosal epithelium only is staged at T3
    E. Mucosal melanoma of the paranasal sinuses are not related to sun exposure

48. **Concerning non-melanomatous skin cancer of the head and neck, which of the following statements is true?**

A. Low-risk, less than 2 cm cutaneous squamous cell carcinoma (SCC) lesions require a 2 mm excision border to give a 95% chance of complete clearance

B. High-risk cutaneous SCC lesions greater than 2 cm in diameter require a 6 mm excision margin

C. All patients with non-melanomatous skin cancer of the head and neck should undergo radiological staging

D. A 3 mm excision margin of a basal cell carcinoma (BCC) gives a 95% of complete resection

E. Parotid involvement in cutaneous SCC (in an N0 neck) requires a radical neck dissection

49. **Concerning cutaneous malignant melanoma, which of the following statements is true?**

A. Require punch biopsy taken from the centre of the lesion for confirmation of the diagnosis

B. The number of mitoses recorded from histopathology is of no prognostic value

C. Patients with stage II cutaneous melanoma require a whole-body (including brain) CT scan

D. Serum lactate dehydrogenase levels directly correlate with survival in stage IV melanoma

E. Cutaneous melanoma having a Breslow thickness of up to 1.0 mm requires a 3 cm excision margin

50. **Anatomy of the skull base: which of the following statements is false?**

A. The maxillary nerve (V2) passes through the foramen rotundum

B. The hypoglossal nerve exits the skull through the hypoglossal canal

C. The lesser wing of the sphenoid is a boundary of the anterior cranial fossa

D. Through the foramen ovale the emissary vein connects the pterygoid plexus with the cavernous sinus

E. The V3 (mandibular nerve) passes through the foramen lacerum

51. **With regard to granulomatous disorders affecting the nose, which of the following statements is true?**

A. Sarcoidosis classically affects the posterior bony septum

B. Syphilis classically affects the nasal mucosa

C. Sarcoidosis classically affects the subglottis

D. The target antigen for perinuclear antineutrophil cytoplasmic antibody (pANCA) is myeloperoxidase

E. Lupus pernio is a cutaneous manifestation of granulomatosis with polyangiitis (GPA)

52. **Concerning congenital midline nasal lesions, which of the following statements is true?**

A. A positive Furstenberg test is associated with an encephalocoele

B. Gliomas enlarge with crying

C. Encephalocoeles are rarely associated with other developmental anomalies

D. Biopsy should be performed in theatre

E. Nasal development occurs at the end of the third trimester

53. **With regard to juvenile angiofibroma, which of the following statements is false?**

    A. The mechanism of bleeding is due to an abnormality of striated muscle within the blood vessel walls
    B. It is associated with familial adenomatous polyposis
    C. It is associated with the Holman–Miller sign on MRI
    D. The tumour arises around the sphenopalatine foramen
    E. Drilling of the basisphenoid at primary surgery helps to reduce recurrence rates

54. **With regard to inverted papilloma, which of the following statements is correct?**

    A. It characteristically arises from the ethmoid sinuses
    B. It has a 20–25% risk of malignant transformation
    C. It is called inverted as the epithelium inverts through the basement membrane
    D. The human papillomavirus (HPV) is implicated in inverted papilloma
    E. On CT it has a classical cerebriform appearance

55. **Regarding antrochoanal polyp, which of the following statements is true?**

    A. It is a common cause of nasal polyposis accounting for 50% of patient who present with nasal polyps
    B. It is commoner in females
    C. It usually occurs in an older population
    D. It is lined by respiratory epithelium with increased inflammatory cells
    E. It responds well to topical nasal steroids as first-line treatment

56. **Regarding orbital cellulitis and cavernous sinus thrombosis, which of the following statements is false?**

    A. The most common organism causing cavernous sinus thrombosis is *Staphylococcal aureus*
    B. The orbital septum is an extension of the periosteum covering bone
    C. Stage III of Chandler's classification involves a subperiosteal abscess
    D. The most common cranial nerve palsy in cavernous sinus thrombosis is a third nerve palsy
    E. The most common cause of cavernous sinus thrombosis is a nasal furuncle

57. **With regard to hereditary haemorrhagic telangiectasia (HHT), which of the following statements is true?**

    A. It features characteristic abnormalities in the clotting studies
    B. It is an autosomal recessive condition
    C. It is due to an abnormality located on chromosome 10
    D. It can be treated with a split skin graft replacing the nasal mucosa
    E. It is diagnosed based on the Radkowski classification

58. **Which of the following reconstructive flaps in the head and neck is correctly matched with their supplying artery?**

    A. Fibula free flap is based on the tibial artery

    B. Pectoralis major flap is based on the thoracoacromial artery

    C. The anterior lateral free flap is based on the popliteal artery

    D. Deltopectoral flap is based on the perforating branches of the internal mammary artery

    E. The supraclavicular flap is based on the external carotid artery

59. **Regarding facial aesthetic analysis, which of the following statements is false?**

    A. The face can be divided vertically into five equal zones with the width of the eye being one fifth.

    B. The nasal labial angle in men should be 90–95 degrees

    C. The nasal facial angle should be approximately 30–40 degrees

    D. The Frankfurt plane is an imaginary line drawn from the inferior portion of the external auditory canal through the superior orbital rim

    E. Goode's method assesses the nasal tip

60. **Regarding nasal tip support mechanisms, which of the following statements is false?**

    A. The medial and lateral crura are major tip support mechanisms

    B. The cartilaginous nasal septum is a minor tip support mechanism

    C. Attachment of the upper lateral cartilages to the lower lateral cartilages is a minor tip mechanism

    D. Attachment of the upper lateral cartilages to the lower lateral cartilages is referred to as the scroll area

    E. Medial crural footplate attachment to the caudal quadrilateral cartilage is a major tip support mechanism

61. **Regarding cerebrospinal fluid (CSF) leak, which of the following statements is true?**

    A. Beta-2 transferrin is associated with a perilymph leak

    B. Spontaneous CSF leaks occur mainly in middle-aged men

    C. CSF is bright on T1 with contrast-weighted MRI scans

    D. The most common site for an iatrogenic injury to the skull base leading to a CSF leak is within the sphenoid

    E. CSF leaks are always associated with meningitis

62. **Regarding disorders of smell, which of the following statements is false?**

    A. In suspected malingering, ammonia is used to test the facial nerve function

    B. They are generally classified into conductive and sensorineural causes

    C. They are common in patients who have had a total laryngectomy

    D. They may be an early sign of Alzheimer's disease

    E. Anosmia is present in Kallmann syndrome

63. **Regarding congenital choanal atresia, which of the following statements is true?**
    A. It is commonly membranous in nature
    B. It most commonly occurs bilaterally
    C. It most often occurs in males
    D. It can be associated with ear abnormalities
    E. It has an incidence of approximately 1:500 live births

64. **Regarding local anaesthesia, which of the following statements is true?**
    A. Lignocaine works by blocking calcium channels
    B. A high pH in the tissues renders the local anaesthetic less effective
    C. The effect of cocaine at preventing monoamine uptake allows it to be an effective local anaesthetic agent
    D. A safe dose of cocaine for nasal surgery is between 1.5 and 3 mg/kg to a maximum dose of 200 mg
    E. Amino ester local anaesthetics are metabolized by the liver

65. **Regarding the ageing face, which of the following statements is true?**
    A. Thinning of the papillary dermis caused by decreased collagen synthesis occurs with ageing in adult life
    B. Ageing is associated with increased subcutaneous fat
    C. Loss of the dermal layer has no effect on skin elasticity and moisture
    D. Prejowel depressions are also known as nasolabial lines
    E. Ultraviolet (UV) exposure does not affect elastin degradation within the dermis

66. **Regarding botulinum toxin, which of the following statements is true?**
    A. Botulinum toxin may be used for focal hyperhidrosis, strabismus, and chronic migraine
    B. It is associated with infection by *Corynebacterium botulinum*
    C. It blocks uptake of acetylcholine in the postsynaptic membrane of nerve endings
    D. It causes permanent muscle paralysis
    E. It causes a similar paralysis to the infection with *Clostridium tetani*

67. **Regarding sutures, which of the following statements is true?**
    A. Vicryl maintains its tensile strength for approximately 42 days
    B. Vicryl is typically absorbed by day 50
    C. Surgical silk is derived from the silkworm species *Bombyx mori*
    D. Silk loses 50% of its tensile strength within 3 months
    E. Nylon loses 15–20% of its tensile strength per year due to absorption

68. **Regarding surgical needles, which of the following statements is true?**
    A. Conventional cutting needles are preferred to reverse cutting needles when closing the pharyngeal mucosa
    B. The reverse cutting needle has its third cutting edge on the inner concave surface
    C. The conventional cutting needle has its third cutting edge on the outer convex surface
    D. Reverse cutting needles are less prone to bending than conventional cutting needles
    E. Cutting needles are preferred for friable tissue

69. **Regarding local anaesthesia to the head and neck, which of the following statements is false?**
    A. The infraorbital nerve can be found in the vertical plane of the pupil 1 cm below the infraorbital rim
    B. The supraorbital nerve can be found in the vertical plane of the pupil at the inferior edge of the supraorbital ridge
    C. The supratrochlear nerve is found at the medial end of the eyebrow
    D. The internal nasal nerve is a terminal branch of the ethmoid nerve that supplies the nasal tip
    E. The mental nerve emerges from the mental foramen 2 cm above the lower border of the mandible along the vertical plane of the pupil

70. **Regarding fungal sinus disease, which of the following statements is true?**
    A. The *Aspergillus* species are most commonly associated with a fungal ball
    B. Allergic fungal sinusitis is not characterized by eosinophilic mucus within the sinuses
    C. *Mucor* species have narrow hyphae with branches at a 45-degree angle
    D. *Aspergillus* species have large, irregularly shaped, non-septate fungal hyphae that branch at right angles
    E. The typical fungal species involved in acute fulminant fungal sinusitis is *Aspergillus*

71. **Regarding chronic rhinosinusitis (CRS), which of the following statements is true?**
    A. The Lund–Mackay scoring system for CRS has a total score of 24
    B. *Staphylococcus aureus* is associated with CRS without nasal polyps
    C. Clarithromycin is the first-line antibiotic of choice in CRS with nasal polyposis
    D. Treatment is guided by a pain scale
    E. The effect of aspirin in Samter's triad is a true allergic response

72. **Regarding mucocoeles and the frontal sinus, which of the following statements is false?**
    A. A mucocoele will demonstrate hyperintensity on T2 MRI
    B. A posterior ethmoid mucocoele may cause orbital apex syndrome
    C. Orbital apex syndrome only involves either or all cranial nerves, III, IV, V1, or VI
    D. Pott's puffy tumour may occur after trauma
    E. The frontal sinuses are not present at birth

73. **A 46-year-old gentleman presents with a 3-month history of right-sided nasal obstruction, pain, bloody rhinorrhoea, and cheek swelling. His CT scan is shown. Which of the following statements is true?**

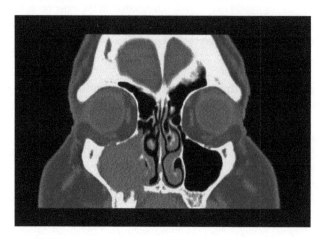

   A. This history and CT scan likely demonstrate chronic rhinosinusitis
   B. Treatment in the UK of this patient would generally follow the EPOS guidelines
   C. There is no bony erosion seen on the scan
   D. This patient should undergo a biopsy and radiological imaging of the neck and chest
   E. Referral back to the general practitioner for a prolonged trial of topical steroids would be appropriate if they had not been trialled

1. D. Allergic fungal sinusitis is characterized by areas of increased attenuation on non-contrast CT. These hyperdense and heterogeneous densities in an opacified sinus are also referred to as the 'double density' sign and most likely represent higher levels of magnesium, manganese, and iron in fungal mucin. The double density sign is also seen in chondrosarcoma, inverted papilloma, and ossifying fibroma.

2. E. Normal ciliary beat frequency is approximately 1000–1500 beats per minute.

The epithelium lining of the upper airways is with ciliated pseudostratified glandular columnar epithelium. There is a 'nine-plus-two' arrangement of the normal cilia, with two central microtubules surrounded by nine microtubule doublets. Nexin arms link the outer doublets. Ciliary movement has an effective stroke phase that sweeps forward and a recovery phase during which the cilia bend backward and extend into the starting position for the stroke phase.

3. D. A endoscopic transethmoidal sphenoidotomy involves an uncinectomy, anterior and posterior ethmoidectomy, before opening the face of the sphenoid inferomedially.

4. D. From the anterior lacrimal crest the anterior ethmoidal artery is approximately 24 mm. The posterior ethmoidal artery is a further 12 mm and the optic nerve a further 6 mm.

5. D. The lateral nasal wall is formed by the bones of the maxilla, palatine, ethmoid, lacrimal, and inferior turbinate.

6. C. The maximum dose of lidocaine without adrenaline is 3–5 mg/kg up to 200 mg. The maximum dose for a 70 kg male is theoretically 350 mg. A solution of 2% lidocaine contains 20 mg/ml.

7. C. Ohngren's line is between the medial canthus and the angle of the jaw. Tumours above this line are associated with a worse prognosis than those below the line.

8. C. In this situation where a CSF leak is highly likely and this is noted at the time of surgery, closure at the primary surgery should be performed. Fluorescein, while used to help with the identification of a CSF leak, is not licensed for this. The consent process should take account of this.

9. D. This is likely to represent a juvenile nasopharyngeal angiofibroma. These are highly vascular benign tumours and therefore a biopsy is not appropriate. Surgery is the treatment of choice and radiotherapy is generally only used for very extensive lesions that cannot be removed surgically or for recurrent disease. Embolization of the sphenopalatine artery may be appropriate.

10. B. Maxillary sinus TNM classification (AJCC).

Primary tumour (T):

- T1: tumour limited to the antral mucosa with no erosion or destruction of bone.
- T2: tumour causing bony erosion or destruction including extension to hard palate and/or middle meatus, except extension to posterior antral wall or pterygoid plates.
- T3: tumour invading any of posterior antral wall, subcutaneous tissues, floor or medial orbit wall, pterygoid fossa, and ethmoid sinuses.
- T4a: tumour invades anterior orbital contents, skin of cheek, pterygoid plates, infratemporal fossa, cribriform plate, sphenoid or frontal sinuses.
- T4b: tumour invades any of orbital apex, dura, brain, middle cranial fossa, cranial nerves other than V(b), nasopharynx, and/or clivus.

11. C. The French catheter scale is used to measure the outside circumference. The diameter (mm) can be calculated by dividing the French size by pi. Therefore a French size 24 equals a diameter of 8 mm.

12. E. Seven bones are considered to make up the bony orbital cavity: the frontal, zygomatic, maxillary, lacrimal, palatine, ethmoid, and sphenoid (greater and lesser wings).

13. C. CSF has a high-intensity signal on T2-weighted imaging and a low-intensity signal on T1-weighted images.

14. E. GPA is characterized by necrotizing granulomas involving the upper respiratory tract, vasculitis of small- and medium-sized vessels, and glomerulonephritis. Untreated, the disease carries a very poor prognosis. The cANCA is more than 90% sensitive and specific for the disease, while 20–40% of cases have raised pANCA.

15. B. The trigeminal nerve supplies innervation to the nose and is sensitive to noxious chemical stimuli, such as ammonia.

16. E. Branchio-oto-renal syndrome is characterized by abnormalities of the ear, branchial clefts, and renal dysplasia.

The frontal sinus originates from pneumatization of the frontal recess into the frontal bone, and is not usually visible at birth. It is usually complete by the age of 20.

The maxillary sinus undergoes two periods of rapid growth associated with dental development (3 years and 7–12 years). Initially the floor of the sinus is above that of the nasal floor, but later it is below the nasal floor.

Prenatal markers for Down syndrome include absent or hypoplastic nasal bones.

Abnormal cilia function is seen in Kartagener syndrome and primary ciliary dyskinesia.

17. C. The Lund–Mackay score is calculated by scoring each sinus complex (maxillary, anterior ethmoids, posterior ethmoids, frontal and sphenoid sinuses) 0–2, where 0 = absence, 1 = partial, and 2 = complete opacification. The osteomeatal complex is scored (0 = clear or 2 = obstructed). A maximum score of 24 is possible.

This series of scans is scored as: right anterior ethmoids = 1; right maxillary sinus = 1; right osteomeatal complex = 2; and left osteomeatal complex = 2 each. Total = 6.

18. D. This unilateral expansile but not erosive mass probably represents an inverted papilloma. It is important initially to establish the diagnosis and then to plan definitive treatment.

19. E. The boundaries of the frontal recess are as follows:

- Medially—middle turbinate
- Laterally—lamina papyracea
- Superiorly—frontal sinus drainage pathway
- Posteriorly—ethmoid bulla
- Anteriorly—agger nasi.

20. D. Hardwood dust is a recognized risk factor for the development of adenocarcinoma of the ethmoid sinuses. The link was first made in High Wycombe, UK, where there was a large number of workers in the furniture industry.

21. B. Asymptomatic nasal septal perforations may simply require nasal hygiene. A large perforation (>2 cm) that causes subjective nasal obstruction, or one which whistles or bleeds, can often be managed with placement of a silastic button. Smaller symptomatic perforations may be amenable to surgical closure with a composite graft of cartilage, perichondrium, and skin, harvested from the pinna.

22. C. Undyed Vicryl might be acceptable, but 2/0 is far too large a suture material in a child's skin. Of the options, Monocryl, an absorbable monofilament material, would give the most acceptable result.

23. C. Performing a 'cephalic shave' will cause cranial tip rotation.

24. B. The nasolabial angle describes the angle between the lip and the caudal end of the nose. This angle describes the degree of nasal tip rotation. The width of the eye is approximately one-fifth of the facial width and is equal to the alar base width and intercanthal distance.

The nasolabial angle is 95–110 degrees in women and 90–95 degrees in men.

Tip projection can be calculated as the ratio of the radix–tip distance tip and the alar–cheek junction distance. In an aesthetically balanced face, this ratio is approximately 0.6.

The face is divided into thirds by horizontal lines drawn adjacent to the menton, alar base, brows, and hairline.

25. C. Nodular melanomas demonstrate predominantly a vertical growth and therefore are considered aggressive.

Tumour thickness, as defined by the Breslow depth, is the most important histological determinant of prognosis. Ulceration is also important and its presence leads to upstaging of the disease.

Superficial spreading melanoma does have an initial radial growth phase followed by a vertical growth phase.

Xeroderma pigmentosa and dysplastic nevus syndrome represent congenital risk factors for developing skin cancers.

Fitzpatrick classified skin types such that type I never tans and always burns. This represents a higher risk than those skins that always tan and never burn.

26. C. The AJCC (2002) uses tumour thickness to stage melanoma. The 2002 AJCC modifications also include histological ulceration and the number of lymph nodes involved rather than size.

Microscopic regional lymph node metastasis as detected by sentinel lymph node biopsy differentiates tumours into those with micro- or macroscopic nodal metastasis.

27. D. The nose has been divided into aesthetic subunits. There are paired lateral nasal wall units, paired alar units, paired soft tissue triangles and single dorsum, tip, and columella subunits.

Burget GC, Menick FJ. Subunit principle in nasal reconstruction. *Plastic and Reconstructive Surgery* 1985;76:239–247.

28. D. A scar that has healed correctly is expected to attain 80% strength compared to normal tissues.

29. E. All of the other answers are associated with an increased risk of developing BCC. Fitzpatrick classified skin types such that type I is fair skin and type VI is black skin. The latter represents a lower risk of developing skin cancer.

30. B. A Z-plasty is used for excising a scar, reorientating, and lengthening a scar. The angle subtended by the arms dictates the lengthening that can be expected.

31. C. The sural nerve has the advantage over the great auricular nerve of having greater length (up to 40 cm) as well as a greater number of neural fascicles. The nerve contains only sensory fibres and lateral foot numbness results after sectioning.

The sural nerve is located between the lateral malleolus and the Achilles tendon, lying deep to the short saphenous vein.

The flexor digiti minimi brevis is supplied by the superficial branch of the lateral plantar nerve.

32. E. During the proliferative phase of wound healing, fibroblasts are attracted by chemotactic factors and begin to arrive on day 3, and peak by day 7.

33. D. Up to four flaps can be designed. Angle * is 60 degrees and angle + 120 degrees. Point d closes to point b. This is a random pattern flap so therefore it is important to consider the distance c to f as the flap receives its blood supply from this pedicle.

34. D. Tumours of the lower lip are squamous cell carcinomas in 98% of cases. There is an overwhelming preponderance of males (ratio 80:1) over females. Clinically apparent cervical metastases are seen in fewer than 10% of patients. Around 5–15% of patients will develop lymph node metastases at some time in the future.

35. E. A full-thickness skin graft relies on its new site for a blood supply. Therefore, any of the options except bare bone would suffice as a recipient site.

36. B. The Abbe lip switch flap is usually used to transfer tissue from the lower to the upper lip. A wedge excision of the upper lip tumour is performed. A wedge of the lower lip is taken, but not completely excised, as the inferior labial artery blood supply is preserved. The lower lip flap is then rotated into the upper lip defect. Three weeks later, the pedicle is divided and the suturing completed.

A dufourmentel flap is similar to a rhomboid flap.

A Karapandzic flap is a bilateral advancement flap extending onto the cheek for lip tumours.

Gillies fan flap is a large rotation flap used for lip tumours.

A radial forearm flap is a free-tissue transfer involving a microvascular anastomosis.

37. C. The sternocleidomastoid flap is a random pattern flap and receives a segmental blood supply from the transverse cervical artery, the superior thyroid artery, and the occipital artery.

38. C. The defect described would have a diameter of 10 mm. Due to the limited quantity and mobility of the skin on the tip of the nose, primary closure is not appropriate. The other methods would be suitable.

39. E. The Abbe flap can be used for defects of the upper or lower lip involving between one-third and two-thirds of the lip. The flap is a two-stage procedure based on the labial artery with division of the pedicle at 2–3 weeks.

40. E. In general, a ratio of 1:2–3 pedicle width to flap length is advised. However, on the face this can often be increased to 1:4–5 due to the excellent blood supply.

A full-thickness skin graft (FTSG) contains the epidermis and the whole of the dermis in contrast to a split-thickness skin graft that contains the epidermis and less than the whole of the dermis. FTSGs do give better cosmetic results.

41. D. The bilobed flap can be used on the nose and exploits the greater skin laxity in other areas to move skin in. The usual angle of rotation is 90–100 degrees. Lobe 1 is usually the width of the defect while lobe 2 is usually narrower. The flap is a stepwise rotational flap. The first lobe should be closed under no tension. The most tension on the wound will be involved in closing the defect formed from lobe 2. The scar is generally complex when closed and this may be a disadvantage cosmetically.

42. E. Moh's micrographic surgery refers to complete micrographic excision of the tumour using intraoperative histopathology to assess for positive margins. This technique is particularly useful for:

- recurrent tumours
- tumours measuring greater than 2 cm
- those with an aggressive histology
- those in cosmetically sensitive areas, since wide excision is often difficult.

43. B. For basal cell carcinoma, a 2–3 mm margin will assure histopathological clearance in 95% of cases.

44. A. Allergies represent type I hypersensitivity reactions as per the Gel and Coombs classification. They are mostly immunoglobulin G (IgE) mediated. There are two major phases for allergic response; the first being the sensitization phase where exposure of the immune system to the allergen causes induction of the IgE antibody; the IgE antibody then binds to mast cells. The second phase is termed the reaction phase; further exposure to the allergen allows binding to the mast cell–IgE antibody complex. Degranulation of the mast cells subsequently occurs causing the release of mediators such as histamine, heparin, proteases, prostaglandins, and kinases. These mediators initiate the symptoms we associate with rhinitis and asthma. The nature and severity of the allergic response varies between individuals and is dependent on the route of exposure and the degree of sensitization; the severest reaction being circulatory collapse associated with anaphylaxis.

The immediate or early phase response to allergy occurs within minutes of exposure to the antigen with vascular permeability and smooth muscle contraction. The late phase typically occurs within 4–8 hours mediated by eosinophils and Th2 helper cells recruited by chemoattractants in the early phase. This phase is generally associated with further smooth muscle contraction and sustained oedema. Corticosteroids generally affect the late phase although there is evidence they may inhibit histamine synthesis.

45. E. During sleep there is muscle relaxation, causing a decrease in tone of the muscles of the upper airway leading to collapse causing obstructive sleep apnoea. This condition would therefore be exacerbated by conditions causing over-relaxation such as alcohol, sleeping tablets, and muscle relaxants. Having a large neck circumference and obesity would be predisposing factors for OSA.

Sleep disorders exist on a spectrum, normal sleep to sleep-disordered breathing, which consists of simple snoring—mild OSA—moderate OSA—severe OSA—obesity hypoventilation syndrome (termed Pickwickian syndrome).

OSA is characterized by recurrent episodes of partial or complete upper airway obstruction during sleep, with the number of episodes per hour determining the severity. The hypoventilation associated with OSA causes hypercapnia and hypoxaemia which stimulate increased respiratory effort. At a certain arousal threshold the patient awakens. This results in a resumption of normal upper airway muscle activity and relief of the upper airway obstruction. Ventilation resumes with correction of the hypercapnia and hypoxaemia. The patient then returns to sleep and the cycle starts again. The hypoventilation and sleep fragmentation associated with this sleep/wake cycle are responsible for the symptoms and the long-term consequences of OSA. Treatment consists of lifestyle advice—weight reduction, alcohol reduction, and correction of medical conditions— anaemia, hypothyroidism. Specifically for OSA, mandibular advancement devices, continuous positive airway pressure (CPAP), and ultimately tracheostomy can be considered. Surgery for snoring may help mild OSA but should not be taken as a specific treatment for OSA. Excision of redundant tissue such as large tonsils may help to reduce the pressures needed for the CPAP device.

46. B. The most common site for nasopharyngeal carcinoma is the fossa of Rosenmuller which is a recess just medial to the medial crura of the Eustachian tube. The aetiology of the condition is thought to be Epstein–Barr virus related, consumption of salted fish containing demethylnitrosamine. Parapharyngeal extension is classified within the T2 category; paranasal sinus involvement would be T3 disease. Non-surgical treatment is the mainstay for nasopharyngeal carcinoma with surgery rarely used for recurrent disease at the primary site or in the neck. Stage 1 and stage 2 disease will receive radiotherapy with stage 3 and stage 4 receiving concurrent chemoradiotherapy. Grommets are rarely used for the middle ear effusion. A hearing aid is advocated in this patient group. Grommet insertion leads to approximately one-third of patients suffering a non-healing perforation and about half of patients will develop troublesome otorrhoea.

47. B. Sinonasal malignant tumours are rare tumours affecting approximately 1:100,000 individuals. The commoner tumours are cancers of epithelial cell origin such as squamous cell carcinoma, adenocarcinoma, olfactory neuroblastoma, adenoid cystic carcinoma, and undifferentiated carcinoma. Olfactory neuroblastomas are thought to arise from the specialized sensory neuroepithelial (neuroectodermal) olfactory cells that are normally found in the upper part of the nasal cavity, including the superior nasal concha, the upper part of the septum, the roof of the nose, and the cribriform plate of the ethmoid. Inverted papilloma is associated with a 2% malignant transformation rate but is also thought to be associated with synchronous SCC of the sinonasal cavity; this potentially increases this figure within the literature. Mucosal melanoma affords a worse prognosis than cutaneous melanoma and thus there is no stage I or II disease, the TNM classification begins at T3.

48. B. Guidelines suggest cutaneous SCC requires a 4 mm excision margin for low-risk lesions with a diameter of 20 mm or less. High-risk lesions with a diameter greater than 20 mm require a 6 mm excision margin. BCC requires a 4 mm excision margin for a 95% chance of tumour clearance. A 3 mm clearance margin in BCC gives an 85% clearance margin. Radiological staging is not routinely performed in cutaneous SCC except when regional lymph nodes are clinically detectable, or because the tumour invades bone. The pattern of spread in cutaneous SCC differs from upper aerodigestive tract mucosal SCC. The parotid and lymph nodes surrounding the external jugular vein, a more superficial lymphatic system, are more likely to be involved. Parotid involvement with an N0 neck dictates a clearance of levels I to III with parotid removal. Parotid involvement and N+ disease requires level V to also be included within the resection.

49. D. As a general rule, all pigmented lesions should be excised with a 2 mm margin and sent for histological analysis. The most important prognostic indictor is tumour depth; this cannot be assessed without the whole lesion being excised. Important prognostic indicators for cutaneous melanoma are depth of invasion (increasing depth means greater likelihood of distant metastases), ulceration, mitotic index, satellite lesions, lymph node involvement, and distant metastases. Stage I and II cutaneous melanoma do not require further investigations. Stage III disease requires CT, head, chest, abdomen, and pelvis and stage IV requires whole-body CT and serum lactate dehydrogenase. The use of PET-CT is also established in melanoma staging assessment as is sentinel lymph node biopsy. Margins are 1 cm for up to 1.0 mm Breslow thickness, 1.01–2 mm thickness requires a 1 to 2 cm excision margin (the added benefit of 2 cm excision over 1 cm has not been proven) but certainly at least a 1 cm excision margin is needed; 2.01 to 4 mm thickness requires a 2–3 cm excision margin (again, there is no absolute proven benefit of 3 cm but at least 2 cm is preferential); and lesions greater than 4 mm Breslow thickness require a 3 cm margin.

50. E. The greater wing of the sphenoid and the lesser wing both are boundaries of the anterior cranial fossa. The lesser wing is a boundary to the posterior aspect and floor of the anterior cranial fossa. Passing through the foramen lacerum are the artery of pterygoid canal, meningeal branch of ascending pharyngeal artery, the occipital artery, and an emissary vein. The nerve of the pterygoid canal passes through its anterior wall.

51. D. Questions regarding granulomatous disorders affecting the upper aerodigestive tract are extremely common in exams. These diseases cause inflammation of the blood vessels and/or impairment of blood flow leading to tissue ischaemia. The common disorders usually examined on are sarcoidosis, GPA (formerly Wegner's granulomatosis), and eosinophilic GPA (formerly known as Churg–Strauss syndrome). Sarcoidosis is a multisystem disease which preferentially affects the lower respiratory tract but may also affect the upper airway, classically supraglottic thickening, and the nasal mucosa—'strawberry skin' which is friable giving crusting, discharge, and nasal congestion. Lupus pernio is a cutaneous manifestation of sarcoidosis. Syphilis classically affects the posterior bony septum. GPA and GPA with eosinophilia are both small- to medium-size vessel vasculitic disorders. GPA classically affects the paranasal sinuses, lungs, and kidneys. The subglottis may be affected. GPA with eosinophilia characteristically has three stages: an allergic phase with asthma and rhinitis, an eosinophilic phase with pneumonia and gastroenteritis, and a vasculitic phase. Antineutrophil cytoplasmic antibodies (ANCA) are antibodies produced by the host against its own proteins. cANCA targets enzyme protease-3 (PR3) present in neutrophil granulocytes, is associated with GPA, and is positive in 95% of those with generalized active disease. pANCA targets the antigen myeloperoxidase (MPO) and is associated with GPA with eosinophilia but can be negative in greater than 50% of cases, being non-specific.

52. A. The crux of the midline nasal lesion lies in understanding embryology.

The critical period for nasal development is the first 12 weeks of fetal development. Failure of this process causes one of the three congenital midline nasal lesions—dermoid, glioma, or encephalocoele. The maxillary processes fuse with the frontonasal processes and the mandibular processes. Failure of this fusion results in a midline defect. There are three key spaces to understand in the embryological development:

- The fonticulus frontalis, the space between the nasal bones and the frontal bones.
- The foramen caecum, located in the anterior cranial fossa, anterior to the cribriform plate of ethmoid bone and posterior to the frontal bone, within the frontoethmoidal suture.
- The prenasal space lies between the nasal bones and the nasal capsule (the precursor to the nasal septum and cartilages).

Nasal dermoids are the most common midline nasal lesion, comprising ectodermal and mesodermal components. They can present as a pit, fistula, or an infected nasal mass anywhere from the glabella to the columella. Hair at the opening is pathognomonic. A central nervous system (CNS) connection is very variable—the literature records 5–50%. Nasal dermoids are associated with other congenital abnormalities but not with syndromes. Complications include infection leading to abscess formation and potential CNS infection. Gliomas are glial tumours found either at the glabella, nasomaxillary suture line, or within the nasal cavity. They can be extranasal or intranasal, with an overall 15% CNS connection. Encephalocoeles are extracranial herniations of meninges (meningoencephalocoeles) and/or brain. These are contiguous with the subarachnoid space. These lesions give a positive Furstenberg test. Encephalocoeles are associated in approximately 40% of cases with other developmental anomalies including microcephaly, hydrocephalus, and agenesis of the corpus callosum. None of the these lesions should be biopsied. Investigations of choice are CT for the delineation of bone and MRI for dural connection and soft tissue analysis.

53. C. This benign and very vascular tumour arises from tissues within the sphenopalatine foramen. It is virtually exclusive to adolescent males; any female presenting with such a tumour would need to undergo chromosomal evaluation. Due to the male preponderance there is much speculation regarding the role of sex hormone receptors in the aetiology of this tumour. Patients with familial adenomatous polyposis have a 25 times higher chance of having one of these tumours compared to the background risk. These tumours are well defined, lobulated, and covered with the mucosa of the nasopharynx. The blood vessels of the tumour lack the smooth muscle and elastic fibres preventing vasospasm.

As the tumour grows it will extend into the nasopharynx, paranasal sinuses, and pterygopalatine and infratemporal fossae. These tumours are locally aggressive. Presentation is usually with recurrent epistaxis and nasal obstruction. Later presentations include cheek swelling, trismus, loss of hearing, anosmia, and eye signs. Following clinical examination, radiological assessment is usually in the form of CT and MRI. Classically on a CT scan, the Holman–Miller sign is seen, referring to bowing of the ipsilateral posterior maxillary wall. Biopsy should generally not be performed—from the patient's demographic information, history, and image studies the diagnosis should be evident.

There are several classification systems including Radkowski, Krouse, and Fisch classifications, which aim to help with treatment options: endoscopic versus open surgery. Treatment is surgical with preoperative embolization. Surgical approaches include endoscopic versus open (transpalatal, lateral rhinotomy, mid-facial degloving, craniofacial resections). The basisphenoid is generally considered the area of recurrence and assessment of this area at primary surgery along with drilling of this bone to ensure residual tumour does not reside within the cancellous bone of the sphenoid or the pterygoid canal greatly improves primary cure rates. Radiation is generally usually reserved for those who are deemed inoperable (generally due to intracranial involvement). Radiotherapy does not offer a cure, mainly reducing tumour bulk, usually giving tumour shrinkage over an extended period of time (2–3 years) with a stabilization of the residual tumour.

54. D. Inverted papillomas are benign epithelial nasal tumours generally arising from Schneiderian epithelium lining of the nasal cavity and paranasal sinuses. They comprise 0.5–4% of all sinonasal tumours removed. The usual presentation is of a unilateral polyp, nasal obstruction, and rhinorrhoea with eventual progression to proptosis. They are benign tumours although they may cause bony destruction as they grow, and have a 2–10% chance of malignant transformation, although malignant transformation is thought to be at the lower end of this percentage, and the higher figure relates to these tumours being associated with a synchronous sinonasal squamous cell carcinoma. Unlike malignant tumours which invade bone, inverted papillomas tend to cause pressure devascularization. Histologically, these tumours demonstrate epithelium which invades the stroma. It is this invagination of epithelium into the surrounding stroma which gives the classical MRI picture of cerebriform (meaning brain-like). (Invasion through the basement membrane is characteristic of carcinoma by definition.)

Treatment is excision either through endoscopic or open approaches. Ideally through an endoscopic approach, a medial maxillectomy is performed affording complete removal of the tumour and allowing greater surveillance in the outpatient setting.

55. D. Antrochoanal polyp is a benign condition usually arising in young adults, typically 25–30 years of age, compared to nasal polyposis which generally occurs with a mean age of presentation at 50 years. One-quarter of patients presenting with an antrochoanal polyp will be children. Antrochoanal polyps account for 4–6% of nasal polyps. There is an equal sex distribution, and although a few studies have found a slight male predominance, they have suffered from small numbers, making this conjecture. The history is characteristically unilateral nasal obstruction and rhinorrhoea. These polyps arise from the maxillary sinus (the posterior wall is generally thought to be the most common place of origin) and extend through a widened ostium into the nasal cavity, and nasopharynx. As for any unilateral nasal lesion CT is usually the investigation of choice, given no bony destruction but a smooth enlargement of the sinus. Treatment is surgical, generally via endoscopic excision. It is important to remove the stalk otherwise there is a potential for recurrence. Histologically, antrochoanal polyps are similar to inflammatory polyps, being lined by respiratory epithelium with increased inflammatory infiltrate, although with much less inflammatory cells and reduced levels of eosinophils compared to nasal polyposis.

56. D. *Staphylococcus aureus* accounts for approximately 70% of cavernous sinus thrombosis. The orbital septum extends from the tarsus to the orbital rim, where it then attaches to the bone and becomes the periorbita inside the orbit and periosteum outside the orbit. Chandler's classification: I, preseptal cellulitis—cellulitis confined to the eyelid (i.e. anterior to the superior orbital septum); II, orbital cellulitis without abscess—cellulitis involving the orbit; III, orbital cellulitis with a subperiosteal abscess; IV, intraorbital abscess; and V, cavernous sinus thrombosis. A sixth nerve palsy is the most common nerve palsy identified in cavernous sinus thrombosis. Cavernous sinus thrombosis most commonly results from contiguous spread of infection from a nasal furuncle (50%), sphenoidal or ethmoidal sinuses (30%), and dental infections (10%).

57. D. Hereditary haemorrhagic telangiectasia (HHT), also known as Osler–Weber–Rendu disease is an autosomal dominant condition. The diagnosis of HHT is made clinically on the basis of the Curaçao criteria. The four clinical diagnostic criteria are:

- epistaxis
- telangiectasias
- visceral lesions
- family history (a first-degree relative with HHT).

This condition affects blood vessels in the skin, mucous membranes, and viscera, causing the classical features of telangiectasia, arteriovenous malformations, and aneurysms, generally occurring in the chest, gut, and brain. The underlying genetic abnormalities are located on chromosomes 9 and 12. Histopathological studies reveal large, irregular, thinly walled blood vessels, but the pathogenesis has not been fully established. Defects in the endothelial cell junctions, endothelial cell degeneration, and weakness of the perivascular connective tissue are thought to cause dilation of capillaries and postcapillary venules, which manifest as telangiectasias. The nasal vessels are particularly prone to bleeding as there is no protective covering layer of squamous epithelium as there is with cutaneous telangiectasia. The clotting studies of these patients are normal.

Management involves gentle packing with adrenaline-soaked packs such as Kaltostat (rather than aggressive nasal packing which will only lead to further trauma and bleeding) and the use of antifibrinolytics (tranexamic acid). These patients have usually undergone multiple blood transfusions, and are generally already treated with ferrous supplementation. Topical oestrogens have been used in management along with coagulative laser (potassium titanyl phosphate (KTP)), septodermoplasty, and Young's procedure.

58. B. The fibula free flap is based on the peroneal artery.

The supraclavicular flap is based on the supraclavicular artery, a branch of the transverse cervical artery; less frequently it arises from the suprascapular artery. Neither are branches of the external carotid artery.

The deltopectoral flap is based on perforating branches of the internal thoracic artery.

The anterior lateral free flap is based on the lateral circumflex femoral artery.

59. D. The Frankfurt plane is an imaginary line drawn from the superior cartilaginous external auditory canal through the infraorbital rim. Goode's method is used to assess projection of the nasal tip and is defined by a line from the nasion to alar groove and a further line from the alar groove to the nasal tip, the ratio of the tip projection to nasal length should be 0.55–0.6 using this method.

60. C. Major tip support mechanisms include the lower lateral cartilages, attachments of the medial crura of the lower lateral cartilages to the caudal septum, and the attachment of the lower lateral cartilages with the upper lateral cartilages (the region termed the 'scroll area').

Minor tip support mechanisms include the soft tissues of the septum, the nasal spine, the soft tissue attachments of the skin and muscle to the alar cartilages, and the nasal dorsum including the dorsal septum and the upper lateral cartilages.

61. A. Beta-2 transferrin is found in CSF and is also found in perilymph. It is not found in blood, mucus, or tears. Spontaneous CSF leaks are twice as likely to develop in women than in men and usually occur in those about 40 years of age. CSF is bright on T2-weighted MRI scans. The most common site for iatrogenic injury is the lateral lamella of the cribriform plate. Management may be conservative or surgical. Generally speaking, if a CSF leak is documented during the endoscopic nasal procedure, it should be formally dealt with at that time. Surgical approaches are endoscopic, extracranial (transfacial incision), and an intracranial or craniofacial approach. The problem with such an approach is retraction of the frontal lobes leading to chronic headaches, potentially seizures, and anosmia.

62. A. In suspected malingering, a noxious stimulus such as ammonia tests the trigeminal nerve. Conductive causes of anosmia include inflammation—rhinosinusitis, polyps, and nasal masses including gliomas and encephalocoeles. Sensorineural causes include vitamin and mineral deficiencies such as zinc and vitamin A; head trauma, which causes shearing of the olfactory nerves; and viral infections. An important sensorineural cause of anosmia is neurological degenerative diseases such as Alzheimer's disease. Kallmann syndrome is caused by failure of the pituitary to release gonadotropin-releasing hormone, preventing the patient entering or completing puberty. Kallmann syndrome differs from other hypogonadotropic hypogonadism disorders due to the associated disorder of smell.

63. D. Congenital atresia occurs in approximately 1:5000 with a female preponderance (2:1 ratio). In approximately 60% of cases the atresia is unilateral. Bony atresia is the most common abnormality either alone or part of a combined bony and membranous atresia. Choanal atresia may be part of the CHARGE syndrome: coloboma, heart abnormality, choanal atresia, retardation of growth, genitourinary anomalies, and ear abnormalities.

64. D. Lignocaine's action is due to the blockage of sodium channels: with sufficient blockage, the membrane of the postsynaptic neuron will not depolarize and the action potential will not be transmitted (they are membrane stabilizers). An acid environment such as within an abscess or inflamed tissue increases the ionization of the local anaesthetic, thus inactivating it by preventing its movement across the cell membrane. The sodium channel blockade gives cocaine its local anaesthetic properties; the blockage of neurotransmission such as monoamine uptake gives cocaine its central effects. There are two groups of local anaesthetics: amino esters and amino amides. Amino esters are metabolized within the plasma via cholinesterases, whereas amino amides are metabolized in the liver.

65. A. The ageing face is due to changes within all layers: skin, fat, muscle, and bone. Ageing is associated with thinner, drier, and less elastic skin. Loss of elastin gives less elastic skin and loss of hyaluronic acid gives the skin less moisture. Loss of subcutaneous fat occurs in the ageing face. Prejowel depressions are also known as marionette lines. Nasolabial folds are known as smile or laughter lines and run from each side of the nose to the corners of the mouth. UV exposure (photoageing) degrades elastin (solar elastosis) within the dermis giving the ageing skin less elasticity.

66. A. Botulinum toxin has many uses in the medical fraternity including within the head and neck. The mechanism of action is blockading the release of acetylcholine from the presynaptic membrane in the nerve endings. The action is temporary with muscle paralysis typically lasting 3 months. Botulinum paralysis is flaccid, the paralysis associated with tetanus infection is spastic; both infections are from *Clostridium* species.

67. C. Vicryl retains its maximal strength for approximately 21 days and complete absorption occurs in 90 days. Nylon loses 15–20% of its tensile strength per year due to hydrolysis.

68. D. With conventional cutting needles the cutting edge is on the inner (concave) surface of the needle. The reverse cutting needle has its third cutting edge on the outer convex surface. This means that conventional cutting needles are associated with cutting through tissue ('cutout'), whereas this problem is not generally associated with reverse cutting needles.

69. D. The supratrochlear nerve is found at the medial end of the eyebrow, 1.5 cm from the midline. The external nasal nerve, a terminal branch of the ethmoid nerve, supplies the nasal tip.

70. A. Acute fulminant fungal sinusitis usually occurs in immunocompromised individuals. *Rhizopus* and *Mucor* species are common causes of this life-threatening condition. Histologically, fungal hyphae can be seen to invade surrounding tissues causing a vasculitis with thrombosis, haemorrhage, and tissue infarction. *Aspergillus* species have hyphae which branch at 45-degree angles. *Aspergillus* species are most commonly associated with a fungal ball (mycetoma). Traditionally, the Bent and Kuhn classification was used to diagnose allergic fungal rhinosinusitis which is associated with eosinophilic-rich mucus.

71. A. The Lund–Mackay scoring system for CRS is based on paranasal CT scans scoring 0 for a clear sinus, 1 for partial opacification, and 2 for completely opacified. Each of the paired maxillary, anterior and posterior ethmoidal, frontal, and sphenoid sinuses is scored, giving a score of 20. Then there is a score for the paired osteomeatal complexes of 0 (unobstructed) or 2 (obstructed), bringing the maximum total score to 24. *Staphylococcus aureus* has been detected in nasal mucus in approximately 70% of patients with CRS with nasal polyps giving rise to the super-antigen theory. Doxycycline is the EPOS 2012 first-line antibiotic for CRS with nasal polyps. Management of CRS is based on a visual analogue scale (VAS) score and nasoendoscopy findings. Diagnosis is based on two or more symptoms persisting for greater than 12 weeks; these symptoms include nasal blockage/obstruction/congestion, nasal discharge (either anterior or posterior nasal drip), facial pain/pressure, and a decrease or loss of smell. Pain in itself would be more typical of an acute sinusitis or another pathology. Serum IgE levels are increased in patients with CRS with nasal polyps. This supports the super-antigen theory. A true allergic response is IgE mediated; Samter's triad, better referred to as aspirin-exacerbated respiratory disease, is a hypersensitivity reaction where the aspirin blocks the cyclooxygenase (COX)-1 enzyme resulting in increased leukotriene levels with the resultant bronchoconstriction.

72. C. Most commonly mucocoeles are hyperintense on T2-weighted MRI scans due to the rich water content. It should be appreciated that colonization with fungus can lead to a very low signal on both T1- and T2-weighted sequences, mimicking a normal aerated sinus. Superior orbital fissure syndrome, whether due to trauma or infection, involves the following structures: cranial nerves III, IV, V1, and VI along with the ophthalmic vein, and sympathetic fibres. The symptoms include ophthalmoplegia, ptosis, ipsilateral forehead paraesthesia, and a fixed dilated pupil. This contrasts with orbital apex syndrome which features the same symptoms, but the involvement of the optic nerve also gives visual change or even blindness. The frontal sinuses usually develop around the age of 2 years and grow further around 6 or 7 years of age and are not completely formed until the early teenage years. Trauma to the frontal sinus drainage system may lead to obstruction and thus infection.

73. D. The scan demonstrates opacification of the right maxillary sinus with erosion of the maxillary floor and potential involvement of the orbit. With this history and scanning in mind, malignancy should be considered until proven otherwise. Other conditions demonstrating a unilateral nature and bone erosion on CT imaging would be fungal disease and inverted papilloma. In this case, the history is more in keeping with malignancy than any other. Chronic rhinosinusitis would not fit the history or imaging.

Section 2

EXTENDED MATCHING QUESTIONS

1. Muscular innervation anatomy

A. Oculomotor nerve
B. Trochlear nerve
C. Trigeminal nerve
D. Abducens nerve
E. Facial nerve
F. Audiovestibular nerve
G. Glossopharyngeal nerve
H. Vagus nerve
I. Accessory nerve
J. Hypoglossal nerve

Which of the nerves listed above provide motor innervation to the following muscles?

1. Orbicularis oculi
2. Cricothyroid
3. Tensor tympani
4. Tensor veli palatini
5. Stylohyoid

2.

A. Sigmoid sinus thrombosis
B. Inhaled foreign body
C. Croup
D. Pendred syndrome
E. Acute epiglottitis
F. Parapharyngeal abscess
G. Retropharyngeal abscess

Match the following radiological sign to the likely pathology from the above list:

1. Steeple sign
2. Widening of pre-vertebral soft tissues
3. Hyperinflated lung on chest X-ray
4. Thumb-printing of epiglottis
5. Delta sign
6. Retropharyngeal abscess

3.

   A. *Clostridium botulinum*

   B. *Staphylococcus epidermidis*

   C. *Streptococcus milleri*

   D. *Pseudomonas aeruginosa*

   E. *Fusobacterium necrophorum*

   F. *Staphylococcus aureus*

   G. *Streptococcus pneumoniae*

   H. *Moraxella catarrhalis*

   I. *Aspergillus fumigatus*

Choose the most likely pathogen from the above list that fits with the following scenario or description:

1. A Gram-positive rod that produces a toxin that blocks neuromuscular blockade
2. A 16-year-old girl with cystic fibrosis presents with a chest infection on the day of surgery
3. A 42-year-old women presenting with a decreased Glasgow Coma Scale score and sepsis. A computed tomography (CT) scan showed a frontal lobe abscess and significant sinusitis
4. A 21-year-old male with a 3-day history of tonsillitis now presents with a temperature, neck pain, and swelling
5. A 16-year-old female presenting with a pinna abscess following an ear piercing through the helix

4. Antibiotics

   A. Beta-lactams

   B. Macrolides

   C. Fluoroquinolones

   D. Tetracyclines

   E. Aminoglycosides

Match the class of antibiotic from the above list with its mechanism of action:

1. Inhibits the activity of DNA gyrase and topoisomerase IV and therefore inhibits cell division
2. Genetic susceptibility to ototoxicity with this drug in people carrying the A1555G mutation
3. Inhibit the cross-linking of peptidoglycans in the cell walls of bacteria

5.

A. Schwannoma
B. Paraganglioma
C. Fibrosarcoma
D. Granulomatosis with polyangiitis
E. Sarcoidosis
F. Chordoma

For each of the following questions, select the most likely histological diagnosis from the list above. Each response may be used once, more than once, or not at all.

1. Following excision of a neck mass, the histology reports a cellular pattern of compact spindle cells (Antoni type A) with more loosely arranged hypocellular zones surrounding it (Antoni B)
2. Following excision of a posterior pharyngeal wall lesion, the histology is reported as showing chronic inflammation, necrosis, granulomas with multinucleated giant cells, vasculitis, and microabscesses
3. Following a postnasal space biopsy, a histopathological report of physaliphorous cells with a 'soap bubble' appearance and compressed nuclei
4. Following a biopsy of neck mass, the report is of a tumour composed of cell nests or 'zellballen' surrounded by sustentacular cells

6.

A. Radicular cyst
B. Ossifying fibroma
C. Fibrous dysplasia
D. Odontogenic keratocyst
E. Ameloblastoma
F. Brown tumour
G. Odontogenic myoxoma
H. Cementoblastoma
I. Central giant cell granuloma
J. Metastatic tumour

For each of the following questions, select the most likely diagnosis from the list above. Each response may be used once, more than once, or not at all.

1. A 15-year-old patient presents with a history of multiple basal cell carcinomas. Which odontogenic lesion should be suspected?
2. A 75-year-old patient is found to have a lesion in her mandible. Biochemical investigations reveal a serum corrected calcium of 3.05 mmol/L (2.12–2.62), phosphate 0.78 mmol/L (0.8–1.45), and parathyroid hormone 262 ng/L (12–72). What is the likely diagnosis?
3. A 14-year-old girl who is under the care of the paediatricians for precocious puberty presents with a unilateral bony swelling over the maxilla. What is the most likely diagnosis?

7.

   A. Bell's palsy
   B. Millard–Gubler syndrome
   C. Mobius syndrome
   D. Ramsey Hunt syndrome
   E. Melkersson–Rosenthal syndrome
   F. Diabetes mellitus
   G. Guillain–Barré syndrome
   H. Lyme disease
   I. Botulism
   J. Syphilis
   K. HIV
   L. Sickle cell disease
   M. Von Recklinghausen's disease

For each of the following situations, select the most likely diagnosis from the list above. Each response may be used once, more than once, or not at all.

   1. A 45-year-old female presents with a severe headache, bilateral facial nerve palsy (House–Brackmann grade III) of 3 days' duration, and a swollen lip. The remainder of the examination was normal

   2. A previously fit and well 45-year-old woman presents a 2-week history of shortness of breath and bilateral facial palsy occurring over the preceding 12 hours. On examination, she has generalized motor weakness and shallow respirations

   3. A 4-year-old child presents with a 3-day history of a left facial nerve palsy and an excoriated region on the left forehead with surrounding erythema, having recently returned from visiting relatives in Australia. The rest of the examination was normal

8.

   A. Apoptosis
   B. Mitosis
   C. Meiosis
   D. Exon
   E. Intron
   F. Codon
   G. Gene
   H. Genome
   I. Messenger RNA
   J. Oncogene
   K. Transcription factor
   L. RNA interference

From the list above, select the correct response to the following questions. Each response may be used once, more than once, or not at all.

   1. The end of which mechanism results in cell death?
   2. What is the name given to the total DNA contained in each cell?
   3. A normally occurring mechanism for the cell to silence specific gene function?

9.

    A. RNA interference
    B. Northern blotting
    C. Southern blotting
    D. Western blotting
    E. cDNA microarray
    F. Polymerase chain reaction (PCR)
    G. Immunohistochemistry
    H. Cell viability assay

For each of the following statements, select the correct technique from the list above. Each response may be used once, more than once, or not at all.

1. A technique for identifying a specific protein in a cell lysate
2. A technique that can assess the expression of many thousands of genes using single-strand oligonucleotides of known sequence
3. A technique for amplifying DNA

10.

    A. Ménière's disease
    B. Syphilis
    C. Cogan's syndrome
    D. Acoustic neuroma
    E. Polyarteritis nodosa
    F. Rheumatoid arthritis
    G. Behçet's syndrome
    H. Systemic lupus erythematosus
    I. Granulomatosis with polyangiitis
    J. Sarcoidosis

Select the condition from the list above that matches each of the following descriptions. Each response may be used once, more than once, or not at all.

1. An autoimmune condition associated with ocular inflammation
2. Associated with progressive sensorineural hearing loss and genital ulceration
3. A condition that may be diagnosed by dark field microscopy

11.

    A. Atrophy
    B. Dysplasia
    C. Hamartoma
    D. Hyperplasia
    E. Hypertrophy
    F. Metaplasia
    G Metastasis
    H. Pleomorphism

For each of the following descriptions, select the correct physiological or pathological process from the list above. Each response may be used once, more than once, or not at all.

1. An increase in the number of cells per unit of tissue
2. A change of one fully differentiated cell into another
3. An increase in the size of individual cells

12.

A. Polyglycolic acid (e.g. Vicryl)
B. Polydioxanone (e.g. PDS)
C. Polycaprone glycolide (e.g. Monocryl)
D. Polypropylene (e.g. Prolene)
E. Silk
F. Braided polyester (e.g. Ethibond)
G. Stainless steel

For each of the following descriptions, select the most likely suture material from the list above. Each response be used once, more than once, or not at all.

1. Induces a local fibrotic reaction, and is degraded by proteolysis over a number of years
2. An example of a synthetic monofilament that maintains tensile strength for many years

13. Types of study

A. Case–control study
B. Cohort study
C. Randomized controlled trial
D. Systematic review
E. Case series study

Which of type of study is best described in the following statements? Each response may be used once, more than once, or not at all.

1. A prospective comparison of two treatments
2. A retrospective study of patients with a disease in an attempt to identify risk factors for that disease
3. A survey to examine the prevalence of a disease
4. A prospective study in which subjects, initially disease free, are followed up

14. Levels of evidence

A. Level 1a
B. Level 1b
C. Level 1c
D. Level 2a
E. Level 2b
F. Level 2c
G. Level 3a
H. Level 3b
I. Level 4
J. Level 5

What level of evidence from the above list is seen in the following types of research? Each response may be used once, more than once, or not at all.

1. Individual randomized controlled trial (RCT)
2. Case series
3. Systematic review (with homogeneity) of RCTs
4. Expert opinion

15.

A. 1 mL
B. 3 mL
C. 25 mL
D. 50 mL
E. 45 mL
F. 90 mL
G. 150 mL

In an average adult male patient, what is the maximum permissible volume from the list above for each of the following drug preparations? Each response may be used once, more than once, or not at all.

1. 0.5% bupivacaine with adrenaline
2. 0.25% bupivacaine with adrenaline
3. Dental Xylocaine®
4. 25% cocaine paste
5. 10% cocaine solution

16.

    A. Chi-square test
    B. Student's t-test
    C. Mann–Whitney U test
    D. McNemar's test
    E. Spearman rank correlation
    F. Logistic regression
    G. Kruskal–Wallis test

What is the most appropriate statistical test from the above list in the following circumstances? Each response may be used once, more than once, or not at all.

1. Input variable and outcome variable are both ordinal
2. Input variable is nominal and outcome variable is non-normal
3. Input variable is nominal and outcome variable is normal
4. Input variable is nominal and outcome variable is quantitative discrete

17.

    A. Standard deviation
    B. Standard error of the mean
    C. Type I error
    D. Type II error
    E. 95% confidence interval
    F. Reference range
    G. Standard error

For each of the following questions, select the correct statistical description from the list above. Each response may be used once, more than once, or not at all.

1. The sample mean plus or minus 1.96 times its standard error
2. Standard deviation/$\sqrt{n}$
3. An estimate of variability of observations
4. A measure of precision of an estimate of a population parameter

18.

    A. Clotting screen
    B. Activated partial thromboplastin time (APTT)
    C. Bleeding time
    D. Factor assays
    E. Genetic screening
    F. Platelet count
    G. A and F
    H. None of the above

For each of the following clinical scenarios, select the most appropriate blood test from the above list. Each response may be used once, more than once, or not at all.

1. A child due to undergo a tonsillectomy with a history of easy bruising and prolonged bleeding from trivial cuts
2. A 55-year-old man, otherwise in good health, admitted to hospital with an uncomplicated nosebleed (first episode) controlled by packing
3. A patient on intravenous heparin for a vascular procedure who develops a profuse nosebleed
4. An alcoholic man admitted with a nosebleed that is slow to respond to first aid

1.

    1. E
    2. H
    3. C
    4. C
    5. E

2.

    1. C

The steeple sign is seen on a frontal neck radiograph. Subglottic tracheal narrowing produces the shape of a church steeple within the trachea. This supports a diagnosis of croup.

    2. G

Widening of pre-vertebral soft tissues suggests a retropharyngeal pathology.

    3. B

A hyperinflated lung on chest X-ray suggests an inhaled foreign body.

    4. E

Thumb-printing of epiglottis indicates a possibility of acute epiglottitis.

    5. A

The empty delta sign is a CT sign of dural venous sinus thrombosis of the superior sagittal sinus, where contrast outlines a triangular filling defect.

3.

    1. A
    2. D
    3. C
    4. E
    5. D

Streptococcus milleri, now known as part of the *Streptococcus anginosus* group, are a group of organisms that are often implicated in head and neck abscess formation and intracranial infections. It is commensal in the oral cavity and oropharynx and can cause significant purulent infection when mucosal barriers are breached.

4.

1. C
2. E
3. A

Penicillins are beta-lactam antibiotics that work by inhibiting bacterial cell wall synthesis by preventing peptidoglycans cross-linking. Quinolones and fluoroquinolones inhibit bacterial replication by blocking their DNA replication pathway. During protein synthesis and DNA replication, the double-stranded DNA needs to unwind, performed by bacterial enzymes called DNA gyrase or DNA topoisomerase. Quinolones and fluoroquinolones inhibit this enzyme by binding to the A-subunit. During this process, bacteria are unable to replicate or even synthesize proteins.

5.

1. A

The histological pattern of alternating regions containing compact spindle cells Antoni type A with more loosely arranged Antoni type regions is characteristic of schwannomas.

2. D

This histopathological description is characteristic of granulomatosis with polyangiitis (formerly Wegener's granulomatosis).

3. F

A chordoma is a tumour of the notochord remnant.

4. B

Paragangliomas are uncommon tumours arising in paraganglion tissue.

6.

1. D

Gorlin syndrome is a rare autosomal dominant condition associated with numerous pathologies including multiple basal cell carcinomas, odontogenic keratocysts, palmar or plantar pits, and bifid, fused, or markedly splayed ribs.

2. F

The patient has primary hyperparathyroidism. Brown tumours (osteoclastomas) are highly characteristic of primary hyperparathyroidism although they may also occur in secondary hyperparathyroidism as well. Brown tumours appear as single or multiple well-circumscribed lesions located within the facial bones as well as the hands, pelvis, and ribs.

3. C

Fibrous dysplasia presents as a painless bony enlargement and is characterized by a ground-glass radiographic pattern. There are two forms. The monostotic form is most common and frequently occurs in the jaws and cranium. The polyostotic form of the disease may be associated with McCune–Albright syndrome (cutaneous pigmentation, autonomic hyper-functioning endocrine glands, and precocious puberty).

7.

1. E

Melkersson–Rosenthal syndrome: the syndrome can present at any age, often with a history of recurrent symptoms that fluctuate in intensity. It is a syndrome consisting of the triad of recurrent lip oedema, recurrent facial paralysis, and a fissured tongue. The changes involved in the lip include episodic non-tender lip swelling which may ultimately become rubbery hard (cheilitis granulomatosa). Only approximately one-third of patients have recurrent facial nerve palsy as part of their syndrome and patients may not present with the complete triad. Other symptoms that may occur include headache, granular cheilitis, trigeminal neuralgia, dysphagia, and laryngospasm.

2. G

Guillain–Barré syndrome is a polyneuropathy affecting the peripheral nervous system, usually triggered by an acute infectious process. The disease is characterized by weakness and paraesthesia affecting the lower limbs first, and progressing in an ascending fashion. The lower cranial nerves may be affected, leading to bulbar weakness.

3. H

Lyme disease: infection with the spirochete *Borrelia burgdorferi* results in Lyme disease. This tick-borne infection is endemic in certain regions of the US as well as Europe and Australia. Facial palsy can occur with infection. Diagnosis is based on serological testing and the treatment is antibiotic therapy.

8.

1. A

Apoptosis is the process of programmed cell death. It is one of the main types of programmed cell death, and involves a series of programmed events.

2. H
3. L

RNA interference is the mechanism by which small double-stranded RNAs can interfere with expression of any mRNA having a similar sequence. The RNAi effect has been exploited by molecular biologists to examining the role of those mRNA messages by their absence.

9.

1. D

This technique is used for analysing mixtures of proteins to show the presence, size, and abundance of one particular type of protein.

2. E

Gene microarray technology has developed with the ability to deposit up to tens of thousands of single-stranded DNA oligonucleotides on a single 'chip'. The different DNA fragments, arranged in such a way that the identity of each fragment is known through its location on the chip, allows the measurement of mRNA expression by hybridizing labelled cDNA to the chip.

3. F

PCR is a technique for replicating a specific piece of DNA *in vitro*.

10.

1. C

Cogan syndrome is thought to be an autoimmune disorder associated with aural symptoms of hearing loss, vertigo and tinnitus, and ocular inflammation

2. G

Behçet syndrome is an autoimmune condition with a triad of oral and genital ulcers, iritis or uveitis, and progressive hearing loss.

3. B

Dark field microscopy involves a special microscope to examine a sample of fluid or tissue from an open sore (chancre) for the spirochetes. If syphilis is present, it can be seen as corkscrew-shaped objects on the microscope slide. This test is used mainly to diagnose syphilis in an early stage.

11.

1. D

Microscopically, cells resemble normal cells but are increased in numbers.

2. F

Transformation of one differentiated cell type to another differentiated cell type.

3. E

Microscopically, cells resemble normal cells but are increased in size.

12.

1. E

Silk is spun by silkworms. Over time the suture becomes absorbed by proteolysis over a number of years. Silk sutures excite an acute inflammatory reaction which leads to encapsulation by fibrous connective tissue.

2. D

This monofilament suture is biologically inert, eliciting minimal tissue reaction. It can maintain tensile strength for up to 2 years.

13.

1. C
2. A
3. E
4. B

14.

1. B
2. I
3. A
4. J

Levels of evidence for studies evaluating therapy, prevention, aetiology or harm:

1a Systematic review (with homogeneity) of RCTs
1b Individual RCT (with narrow confidence interval)
1c All or none
2a Systematic review (with homogeneity) of cohort studies
2b Individual cohort study (including low-quality RCT; e.g. <80% follow-up)
2c 'Outcomes' research
3a Systematic review (with homogeneity) of case–control studies
3b Individual case–control study
4 Case-series (and poor-quality cohort and case–control studies)
5 Expert opinion without explicit critical appraisal, or based on physiology, bench research, or 'first principles'

15.

1. E
2. F
3. C
4. A
5. B

Drug volume calculations:

0.1% = 1 mg/mL = 1:1000

1% = 10 mg/mL = 1:100

10% = 100 mg/mL = 1:10

Maximum drug doses:

- Lignocaine, maximum dose:
  - Plain = 300 mg
  - With adrenaline = 500 mg
- Bupivacaine, maximum dose:
  - Plain = 175 mg
  - With adrenaline = 225 mg
- Cocaine, maximum dose: 200 mg.

Calculations for question 14:

1. 0.5% bupivacaine with adrenaline:

Maximum dose = 225 mg

[bearing in mind that 0.5% bupivacaine = 5 mg/mL]

Maximum dose = 225/5 = 45 mL.

2. 0.25% bupivacaine with adrenaline:

Maximum dose = 175 mg

[bearing in mind that 0.25% bupivacaine = 2.5 mg/mL]

Maximum dose = 175/2.5 = 90 mL.

3. Dental Xylocaine® = 2% lignocaine + 1:80,000 adrenaline:

Maximum dose = 500 mg

[bearing in mind that 2% lignocaine = 20 mg/mL]

Maximum dose = 500/20 = 25 mL.

4. 25% cocaine paste:

Maximum dose = 200 mg

[bearing in mind that 25% cocaine = 250 mg/mL]

Maximum dose = 200/250 ≈ 1 mL.

5. 10% cocaine solution:

Maximum dose = 300 mg

[bearing in mind that 10% cocaine solution = 100 mg/mL]

Maximum dose = 300/100 = 3 mL.

Table 6.1 Outcome variable

Input variable	Nominal	Categorical (>2 categories)	Ordinal	Quantitative discrete	Quantitative non-normal	Quantitative normal
Nominal (e.g. treatment vs placebo)	χ^2 or Fisher's	χ^2	χ^2 trend or Mann–Whitney	Mann–Whitney	Mann–Whitney or log-rank (a)	Student's t-test
Categorical (>2 categories)	χ^2	χ^2	Kruskal–Wallis (b)	Kruskal–Wallis (b)	Kruskal–Wallis (b)	Analysis of variance (c)
Ordinal (ordered categories)	χ^2-trend or Mann–Whitney	(e)	Spearman rank correlation	Spearman rank correlation	Spearman rank correlation	Spearman rank correlation or linear regression (d)
Quantitative discrete	Logistic regression	(e)	(e)	Spearman rank correlation	Spearman rank correlation	Spearman rank correlation or linear regression (d)
Quantitative non-normal	Logistic regression	(e)	(e)	(e)	Plot data and Pearson or Spearman rank correlation	Plot data and Pearson or Spearman rank correlation and linear regression
Quantitative normal	Logistic regression	(e)	(e)	(e)	Linear regression (d)	Pearson and linear regression

16.

1. E
2. C
3. B
4. C

Choice of statistical test for independent observations:

(a) If data are censored.

(b) The Kruskal–Wallis test is used for comparing ordinal or non-normal variables for more than two groups, and is a generalization of the Mann–Whitney U test. The technique is beyond the scope of this book, but is described in more advanced books and is available in common software (Epi-Info, Minitab, SPSS).

(c) Analysis of variance is a general technique, and one version (one-way analysis of variance) is used to compare normally distributed variables for more than two groups, and is the parametric equivalent of the Kruskal–Wallis test.

(d) If the outcome variable is the dependent variable, then provided the residuals are plausibly normal, then the distribution of the independent variable is not important.

(e) If data are censored.

(f) There are a number of more advanced techniques, such as Poisson regression, for dealing with these situations. However, they require certain assumptions and it is often easier to either dichotomize the outcome variable or treat it as continuous.

17.

1. E
2. B
3. A
4. G

The standard error of the mean of one sample is an estimate of the standard deviation that would be obtained from the means of a large number of samples drawn from that population.

A standard deviation is a sample estimate of the population parameter; that is, it is an estimate of the variability of the observations.

A standard error, on the other hand, is a measure of precision of an estimate of a population parameter.

18.

1. D

This scenario suggests a coagulopathy or thrombocytopenia. Factor assays may be required if the clotting screen is abnormal.

2. H

In this situation, no specific tests of clotting are required.

3. B

The APTT is used to monitor heparin therapy. If excessively prolonged, epistaxis may occur.

4. G

Alcoholic patients are more likely to have derangement of liver function, causing reduction in clotting factors and low platelet count.

1.

A. Sural interposition graft
B. Fascia lata sling
C. End-to-end anastomosis
D. Botox
E. Hypoglossal facial anastomosis

When considering facial nerve reanimation, which treatment from the above list is the most appropriate for the following situations?

1. A 34-year-old lady with a longstanding facial nerve palsy following a Bell's palsy who now complains of synkinesis
2. A 55-year-old man who sustained a complete facial nerve palsy post cerebellopontine angle surgery 6 months ago
3. A 70-year-old lady complaining of drooling with a 2-year history of complete facial nerve palsy following a malignant parotid lesion
4. A 45-year-old lady with a complete facial nerve palsy following a gunshot wound
5. A 16-year-old boy with a complete facial nerve palsy following temporal bone fracture and transection in the vertical segment of the nerve

2.

A. Tympanomastoid suture line
B. Osseocartilaginous junction
C. Between jugular foramen and the carotid canal
D. Fissures of Santorini
E. Petrotympanic fissure

Match each of the following descriptions with a structure listed above:

1. Commonly find osteomas here
2. The chorda tympani runs in this
3. Erosion here is called Phelp's sign
4. Connects the parotid to the lateral external auditory canal
5. Exostoses are commonly found here

3.

A. Probable Menière's disease
B. Tumarkin crisis
C. Cochlear hydrops
D. Delayed endolymphatic hydrops
E. Lermoyez syndrome

Match each of the options in the above list with the following statements:
1. A 35-year-old male with increasing tinnitus, hearing loss, and fullness relieved by a spell of vertigo
2. A 50-year-old male with sudden loss of extensor function causing a drop attack
3. A 40-year-old female with hearing loss, tinnitus, and aural fullness
4. Two episodes of vertigo lasting 45 minutes with patient awareness of hearing loss after the episode
5. A 40-year-old with longstanding sensorineural hearing loss and recent onset of vertigo with tinnitus

4.

A. Waardenburg syndrome (type 4)
B. Waardenburg syndrome (type 2)
C. Usher syndrome
D. Pendred syndrome
E. Alport syndrome

Match each of the following scenarios with the most appropriate diagnosis from the list above:
1. Patient presents with sensorineural hearing loss and Hirschsprung's disease
2. Patient presents with sensorineural hearing loss and progressive visual loss
3. Patient presents with sensorineural hearing loss and no dystopia canthorum
4. Patient presents with sensorineural hearing loss and retinal flecks
5. Patient is found to have an associated enlarged vestibular aqueduct

5.

A. Left-beating horizontal nystagmus
B. Right-beating horizontal nystagmus
C. Vertical nystagmus with downward gaze
D. Right geotropic nystagmus
E. Left geotropic nystagmus

Match the nystagmus from the list above with the following scenarios:
1. Spinning on a merry-go-round in a clockwise direction resulting in ampullopetal stimulation to the left lateral squamous cell carcinoma (SCC)
2. During caloric testing, 30°C water is administered to the left ear
3. A positive Dix–Hallpike test in a left posterior canal benign paroxysmal positional vertigo
4. Removal of cholesteatoma matrix from a right lateral SCC resulting in severe perilymph leak which cannot be controlled
5. Positive fistula test in a patient with a right lateral SCC dehiscence

6.

    A. Type As
    B. Type Ad
    C. Type B
    D. Type C
    E. Type D

Match each of the following conditions with their likely respective tympanogram from the above list:

1. Extensive tympanosclerosis with a small anterior tympanic membrane perforation
2. Extensive tympanosclerosis with an intact tympanic membrane
3. A tympanic membrane clinically showing Schwartz's sign
4. Temporal bone fracture with a maximal conductive hearing loss and clinical appearance of a dislocated incudostapedial joint
5. A patient with intermittent sensation of muffled hearing and occasional ability to autoinflate her ears

7.

    A. Visual reinforcement audiometry
    B. Play audiometry
    C. Pure tone audiometry
    D. Otoacoustic emissions

From the list above, choose the most appropriate subjective hearing test for the following children:

1. A developmentally normal 3-year-old child
2. A developmentally normal baby
3. A developmentally normal 12-month-old infant

8.

    A. Computed tomographic (CT) scan with intravenous (IV) contrast
    B. Positron emission tomographic (PET) scanning
    C. Angiography
    D. T2-weighted magnetic resonance imaging (MRI)
    E. MRI with IV contrast
    F. High-resolution CT scan without contrast
    G. Diffusion-weighted MRI

Choose the optimum imaging modality from the list above in each of the following situations:

1. A 45-year-old lady with asymmetric sensorineural hearing loss and unilateral tinnitus
2. A 19-year-old male who underwent combined approach tympanoplasty 12 months ago for cholesteatoma. He had problems post anaesthetic and would prefer to avoid the second-look surgery originally planned for him
3. A 30-year-old male who has haemotympanum and facial palsy following a road traffic collision

9.

    A. Recreates the antihelix by anterior scoring of auricular cartilage
    B. Recreates the antihelix with permanent horizontal mattress sutures
    C. Recreates the antihelix by incising the cartilage and placing buried mattress sutures
    D. Classically involves complete transection of auricular cartilage
    E. Uses a diamond burr to recreate the antihelix

Link each of the following eponyms with the pinnaplasty technique described above:
    1. The Mustarde technique
    2. The Converse technique
    3. The Stenstrom technique
    4. The Weerda technique

10.

    A. Cogan syndrome
    B. Alport syndrome
    C. Apert syndrome
    D. Refsum syndrome
    E. Down syndrome
    F. Crouzon syndrome
    G. Treacher Collins syndrome
    H. Pendred syndrome

Select the syndrome from the list above that corresponds with the following clinical findings:
    1. Sensorineural hearing loss and renal abnormality
    2. Sensorineural hearing loss and interstitial keratitis
    3. Conductive hearing loss, deformed pinnae, and retrognathia
    4. Sensorineural hearing loss and need for thyroxine treatment

11.

    A. The first branchial arch
    B. The second branchial arch
    C. The otic capsule
    D. The second branchial arch and the otic capsule
    E. The first branchial arch and the otic capsule
    F. The first and second branchial arches

The following inner ear structures develop from which of the list above?
    1. The stapes bone
    2. The malleus bone
    3. The incus bone

12.

 A. Schwartze's sign (reddish hue of the tympanic membrane)

 B. Brown's sign (blanching of the tympanic membrane on pneumatic otoscopy)

 C. Hennebert's sign (ocular deviation with pneumatic otoscopy)

 D. Paracusis Willisii (apparent improvement in hearing for conversation against background noise)

 E. Diplacusis (apparent difference in pitch of a tone perceived by both ears)

 F. Oscillopsia

 G. Brun's sign (intermittent headache, vertigo, and vomiting)

 H. Hitselberger's sign (reduced sensitivity over the posterosuperior aspect of the concha)

 I Griesinger's sign (oedema and tenderness over the mastoid cortex)

For each of the following diagnoses, select the most likely sign from the list above. Each response may be used once, more than once, or not at all.

 1. Which sign is likely to be positive in a patient diagnosed with otosyphilis?

 2. Which sign may be positive in a patient with pulsatile tinnitus?

 3. Which sign may be present in a patient with an acoustic neuroma?

13.

 A. [Bracket open to the right

 B.] Bracket open to the left

 C. Δ Triangle

 D. Circle, unfilled

 E. Circle, filled

 F. Arrow

 G. |

 H.]

For each of the following questions, select the correct audiological symbol from the list above. Each response may be used once, more than once, or not at all.

 1. According to the British Society of Audiology, which symbol represents unmasked bone conduction?

 2. According to the British Society of Audiology, which symbol represents left-sided uncomfortable loudness levels?

 3. According to the British Society of Audiology, which symbol represents right air conduction?

14.

    A. Behind-the-ear (BTE)

    B. Bone-conduction hearing aid

    C. Bone-anchored hearing aid (BAHA)

    D. In-the-ear (ITE)

    E. Vented mould behind-the-ear

    F. Body-worn hearing aid

    G. Cochlear implant

For each of the following situations, select the most appropriate initial hearing aid from the list above. Each response may be used once, more than once, or not at all.

1. A child of 5 years of age with a profound bilateral hearing loss
2. An adult with Down syndrome with persistently discharging ears and a conductive hearing loss
3. An 80-year-old lady with severe rheumatoid arthritis who lives alone
4. A 30-year-old solicitor with a mild low-tone sensorineural hearing loss

15.

    A. Dexamethasone, neomycin, acetic acid

    B. Dexamethasone, framycetin, gramicidin

    C. Hydrocortisone, gentamicin

    D. Triamcinolone, gramicidin, neomycin, nystatin

    E. Hydrocortisone, neomycin, polymixin B

    F. Clotrimazole

What active ingredients are in the following ear medications? Each response from the list above may be used once, more than once, or not at all.

1. Otosporin
2. Tri-adcortyl otic
3. Sofradex
4. Otomize
5. Canesten

16. Examine the following trace of an auditory brainstem response (ABR)

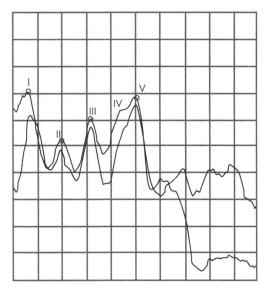

A. Cochlea
B. Cochlear nerve
C. Cochlear nucleus
D. Olivary complex
E. Lateral lemniscus
F. Corona radiata
G. Auditory cortex
H. Inferior colliculus

For each of the following waves, select the correct structure from the list above that is responsible for each peak on the ABR trace. Each response may be used once, more than once, or not at all.

1. Wave III
2. Wave IV
3. Wave V
4. Wave I

1.

   1. D

Synkinesis can be effectively treated with Botox.

   2. E

Hypoglossal facial anastomosis is an effective treatment for facial nerve palsy where end-to-end and cable grafting is not possible. Patients can expect their facial nerve function to improve to House–Brackman grade 3 at best.

   3. B

The extended period of time this lady has had a facial nerve palsy means that the motor end plates are likely to have atrophied. Dynamic techniques will be ineffective and a static technique is appropriate here.

   4. A

Gunshot wounds are likely to preclude end-to-end anastomosis and require an interposition graft. A sural interposition graft is suitable; if trauma has not occurred around the neck, the greater auricular nerve may also be used.

   5. C

Following exploration, a nerve transection in the vertical segment can usually be repaired with an end-to-end anastomosis. Nerve rerouting can help approximate nerve endings.

2.

   1. A

Osteomas are usually found in the tympanomastoid or tympanosquamous suture line.

   2. E

The chorda tympani branches off the facial nerve in its vertical segment. It crosses the middle ear passing between the malleus and incus on the medial surface of the neck of malleus. It exits the middle ear through the petrotympanic fissure also known as Glaserian fissure along with the anterior tympanic branch of the internal maxillary artery.

   3. C

Phelp's sign is erosion of the caroticojugular spine between the carotid canal and jugular fossa found in glomus jugulare tumours.

   4. D

Fissures of Santorini are vertical fissures in the anterior portion of the external auditory canal that give more flexibility to the external canal but also allow infection and tumour to spread between the external auditory canal and the parotid gland.

   5. B

Exostoses commonly form at the tympanic ring or osseocartilaginous junction of the ear canal.

3.

1. E

Lermoyez syndrome is a rare variant of Ménière's with hearing improvement and reduction of tinnitus during vertiginous attacks.

2. B

A Tumarkin crisis is poorly understood but thought to be caused by a sudden severe misfiring of the otolithic organ causing the patient to fall suddenly. Usually, they occur frequently for less than a year before spontaneous remission.

3. C

Cochlear hydrops is thought to be an early form of Ménière's that spares the vestibular system.

4. A

The diagnostic criteria for Ménière's changed in 2015. The new guidelines state that definite Ménière's must have two or more spontaneous episodes of vertigo, lasting 20 minutes to 12 hours, with audiometrically documented low-to-medium sensorineural hearing loss, fluctuating aural symptoms (hearing, tinnitus, or fullness) and no better diagnosis. Probable Ménière's is defined as two or more episodes of vertigo or dizziness, each lasting 20 minutes to 24 hours with fluctuating aural symptoms (hearing, tinnitus, or aural fullness) and no better diagnosis.

5. D

Delayed endolymphatic hydrops is a term coined by Schuknecht which describes the subset of patients who have sustained profound hearing loss and then after a prolonged period of time develop either episodic vertigo in the same ear.

4.

1. A

Waardenburg syndrome type 4 is an autosomal dominant condition characterized by hearing loss, pigmentation to the hair, skin, and eyes; and Hirschsprung's disease. It can be further divided into 4A, 4B, and 4C.

2. C

Usher syndrome is an autosomal recessive condition characterized by sensorineural hearing loss and progressive visual loss due to retinitis pigmentosa. It is divided into type 1, 2, and 3 distinguished by severity.

3. B

Waardenburg syndrome type 2 is an autosomal dominant condition characterized by varying degrees of deafness and pigmentation. It is differentiated from type 1 by the absence of dystopia canthorum.

4. E

Alport syndrome is a variably inherited condition characterized by kidney disease, hearing loss, and eye abnormalities including anterior lenticonus (cone-shaped lens) and retinal flecks.

5. D

Pendred syndrome is an autosomal recessive condition characterized by sensorineural hearing loss and euthyroid goitre. It can cause balance problems and is commonly associated with an enlarged vestibular aqueduct and cochlea hypoplasia.

5.

1. A
2. B
3. E
4. A
5. B

Irritative nystagmus will cause ipsilateral nystagmus, as opposed to paralytic which will cause contralateral nystagmus. The mnemonic 'COWS' (cold opposite, warm same) aids in remembering caloric test outcomes in normally functioning canals. It is important to remember that perilymph flow in the lateral semicircular canals toward the ampulla (ampullopetal) is stimulatory, whereas flow away from the ampulla (ampullofugal) reduces stimulation; note that this is contrary to the other semicircular canals where the opposite is true. The nystagmus of benign paroxysmal positional vertigo is torsional, geotropic, latent, and fatiguing.

6.

1. C
2. A
3. A
4. B
5. D

Tympanometry is a non-behavioural test of middle ear function. The horizontal axis shows negative, neutral, and positive air pressure measured in either mm H_2O or decapascals (daPa). The vertical axis shows compliance from minimum at the bottom to maximum towards the top and is often designated in millilitres (mL). Type A tympanogram represents a normal middle ear pressure and thus tympanic membrane (TM) compliance, though it is worth remembering that these may be subdivided into a tympanogram with abnormally high static compliance (Ad), or an abnormally low compliance (As). A Type B tympanogram (flat trace) occurs when no air pressure change in the outer ear canal results in no TM compliance, whereas type C traces represent negative middle ear pressures. With this information, the correct corresponding tympanograms are relatively easy to establish. Type D does not exist.

7.

1. B
2. D
3. A

Visual reinforcement audiometry is a subjective hearing test appropriate for infants from 6 months to 2 years old. It involves conditioning the child to sound with the visual reward of an illuminated toy or puppet. Tones or warbles are then presented at reducing intensity until the minimum response level is ascertained.

Play audiometry is a subjective test of hearing for children who can understand simple instructions and commands. This would include developmentally normal children between the ages of approximately 2 and 5 years. It involves a game in which the child performs an action (typically putting toy figures in a boat) when a sound is heard. Various frequency sounds are presented to the child in reducing volume to determine the threshold.

Pure tone audiometry is a subjective test of hearing which is appropriate for school-age children (approximately 4 years and upwards), although some younger children may also be able to manage this test.

Otoacoustic emissions are used as an objective test of hearing where sound is presented to the ear canal using a probe. When the sound stimulates the hair cells in the cochlea, the outer hair cells twitch in response, creating echo which is picked up by a microphone situated in the probe. This forms the cornerstone of the newborn hearing screening programme.

8.

1. E
2. G
3. F

In situation 1, an acoustic neuroma is suspected. The imaging modality of choice is contrast-enhanced MRI on T1-weighted images.

In situation 2, the patient wishes to avoid surgery, so the modality of choice for detecting any recurrent cholesteatoma would be diffusion-weighted MRI. However, this will only detect recurrences of 2–3 mm in diameter.

In situation 3, a temporal bone fracture is suspected. High-resolution CT would be the optimum choice for bony definition and determining if the facial nerve has been impinged or divided.

9.

1. B
2. D
3. A
4. E

The Stenstrom technique recreates the antihelix by anterior scoring of auricular cartilage.

The Mustarde technique recreates the antihelix with permanent posterior horizontal mattress sutures.

The Converse technique classically involves complete transection of auricular cartilage.

The Weerda technique uses a diamond burr to recreate the antihelix.

10.

1. B
2. A
3. G
4. H

Both Alport and Cogan syndromes are associated with sensorineural hearing loss. Interstitial keratitis is found in Cogan syndrome, whereas renal abnormalities are typical of Alport syndrome.

Patients with Treacher Collins syndrome typically have conductive hearing loss and characteristic facial features including downslanting palpebral fissures, deformed pinnae, and retrognathia.

Pendred syndrome combines sensorineural hearing loss with goitre. Patients can be euthyroid or hypothyroid.

11.

   1. D
   2. F
   3. F

The ossicles develop from the first and second arch cartilages, and the otic capsule. The head of malleus and body of incus develops from the first arch (Meckel's cartilage). The handle of malleus, long process of incus, and crurae of stapes develop from the second arch (Reichert's cartilage). The foot plate of the stapes develops from the otic capsule.

12.

   1. C

Hennebert's sign (ocular deviation with pneumatic otoscopy). This may also be positive in a patient with superior semicircular canal dehiscence. It is thought to be due to a fibrous band between saccule or utricle resulting in vestibular stimulation with footplate movement and greater with negative pressure.

   2. B

Brown's sign (blanching of the tympanic membrane on pneumatic otoscopy) is seen in those patients with a glomus tympanicum tumour.

   3. H

Hitselberger's sign. Due to a pressure effect on the facial nerve in the internal auditory meatus.

13.

   1. C
   2. H
   3. D

14.

   1. A
   2. B

Although this adult with Down syndrome may eventually require a BAHA, his most appropriate initial hearing aid would be a bone-conduction hearing aid.

   3. F

An elderly arthritic lady is unlikely to be able to manipulate the controls of a conventional BTE aid.

   4. D

For a mild low-tone loss in a young professional, an ITE or in-the-canal (ITC) aid might be appropriate.

15.

   1. E
   2. D
   3. B
   4. A
   5. F

16.

1. D
2. E
3. H
4. B

The mnemonic to remember ABR waves is:

I   E: Eighth nerve action potential
II C: Cochlear nucleus
III O: Olivary complex
IV L: Lateral lemniscus
V   I: Inferior colliculus
VI Medial geniculate
VII Auditory radiation (Brodmann's area 41)

1.

A. Chronic lymphocytic thyroiditis (Hashimoto's disease)
B. Invasive fibrous thyroiditis
C. Lymphoma
D. Microbial inflammatory
E. Papillary cell carcinoma thyroid
F. Parapharyngeal abscess
G. Subacute granulomatous thyroiditis
H. Subacute lymphocytic thyroiditis
I. Tonsillitis

Please look at the following patient scenarios and match the most likely diagnosis from the list above. Each response can be used once, more than once, or not at all.

1. A 30-year-old female, with a past medical history of Sjögren syndrome presents with a firm, non-tender goitre and positive antithyroid microsomal antibodies
2. A 28-year-old female, 3 months postpartum, presents with tachycardia, palpitations, white cell count is normal, T4 is increased, and thyroid-stimulating hormone decreased
3. A 50-year-old female presents with an acutely tender neck, worse on neck movement. She has raised inflammatory markers and an increased T4 and thyroglobulin levels

2.

A. Chronic hyperplastic candidosis
B. Denture stomatitis
C. Gingival hyperplasia
D. Major aphthous ulceration
E. Oral candidiasis
F. Oral lichen planus
G. Proliferative verrucous leucoplasia
H. Systemic lupus erythematosus (SLE)
I. Squamous cell carcinoma
J. Traumatic ulceration

For each of the following scenarios, please choose the most likely diagnosis from the list above. Each response can be used once, more than once, or not at all.

1. A 50-year-old male patient presents to a head and neck follow-up clinic following transoral resection of a tonsil tumour with a 4-week history of a well-defined ulcer on the lateral border of his tongue

2. A 45-year-old male presenting with a large, non-homogeneous leucoplastic area on his buccal mucosa

3. A 60-year-old female presents with multiple raised white lesions within her oral cavity

4. A 70-year-old male presenting to the head and neck follow-up clinic with an erythematous area, demarcated by his upper denture

5. A 64-year-old female with known hypertension on amlodipine presents with ill-fitting dentures

6. Oral ulceration associated with bilateral parotid gland enlargement and facial rash

3.

    A. Acinic cell carcinoma

    B. Basal cell adenoma

    C. Cribriform adenoid cystic carcinoma

    D. High-grade mucoepidermoid carcinoma

    E. Melanoma

    F. Low-grade mucoepidermoid carcinoma

    G. Oncocytoma

    H. Papillary cystadenoma lymphomatosum

    I. Pleomorphic adenoma

    J. Salivary duct carcinoma

    K. Solid form adenoid cystic carcinoma

    L. Squamous cell carcinoma

    M. Thyroglossal cyst

Please match each of the following the histories to the most likely diagnosis from the list above. Each response can be used once, more than once, or not at all.

1. A 70-year-old male presents with a rapid onset of a 3 cm swelling in the tail of his left parotid. He has a left-sided grade III House–Brackmann facial palsy. Histology reveals pleomorphic tumour cells with a cribriform pattern

2. A 40-year-old female presents with a mass in her right parotid; histology following excision notes a large number of mucin containing cells

3. A 45-year-old female with a right submandibular mass. Following excision, histology reveals nests of cells in microcystic spaces with perineural invasion

4.

    A. Foramen ovale

    B. Foramen rotundum

    C. Superior orbital fissure

    D. Inferior orbital fissure

    E. Internal acoustic meatus

    F. Foramen magnum

    G. Jugular foramen

    H. Pterygoid canal (vidian canal)

    I. Hypoglossal canal

    J. Petrotympanic fissure (Glaserian fissure)

    K. Foramen spinosum

    L. Olfactory groove

Select the correct foramen from the list above for each of the following descriptions. Each response may be used once, more than once, or not at all.

1. The spinal accessory nerve exits through it

2. The lesser petrosal nerve exits through it

3. The chorda tympani enters the infratemporal fossa through it

5.

    A. Deltopectoral flap

    B. Midline forehead flap

    C. Temporalis flap

    D. Pectoralis major flap

    E. Latissimus dorsi flap

    F. Trapezius flap

    G. Sternocleidomastoid flap

    H. Radial forearm flap

    I. Scapular flap

    J. Rectus abdominus flap

    K. Lateral thigh flap

From the list above, select the correct flap corresponding to the following questions. Each response may be used once, more than once, or not at all.

1. Which fasciocutaneous flap is based on the first four perforating branches of the internal mammary artery?
2. Which flap receives a segmental blood supply which includes the transverse cervical artery?
3. Which flap is unlikely to be available in a patient with Poland syndrome?

6.

    A. Vidian nerve

    B. Facial nerve

    C. Greater superficial petrosal nerve

    D. Lingual nerve

    E. Hypoglossal nerve

    F. Descendens hypoglossi nerve

    G. Lesser petrosal nerve

For each of the following descriptions, select the correct nerve from the above list. Each response may be used once, more than once, or not at all.

1. Supplies only parasympathetic innervation to the nose
2. Contributes to the ansa cervicalis
3. Supplies parasympathetic innervation to the parotid gland
4. It is the continuation of Jacobsen's nerve
5. It is a branch of the glossopharyngeal nerve

7.

   A. Mucoepidermoid carcinoma
   B. Carcinoma ex pleomorphic adenoma
   C. Adenocarcinoma
   D. Adenoid cystic carcinoma
   E. Acinic cell carcinoma
   F. Squamous cell carcinoma
   G. Basaloid carcinoma
   H. Rhabdomyosarcoma

For each of the following clinical scenarios, select the most likely diagnosis from the list above. Each response may be used once, more than once, or not at all.
1. A 45-year-old woman with a firm lesion on the hard palate and lung metastases
2. A 70-year-old man with a longstanding parotid mass that then begins to enlarge rapidly
3. A 67-year-old smoker with a firm lesion on his lower lip
4. A 50-year-old woman with salivary gland malignancy and trigeminal symptoms

8.

   A. KTP
   B. CO_2
   C. Pulsed dye
   D. Holmium
   E. Argon
   F. Helium–neon

For each of the following statements, select the correct type of laser from the list above. Each response may be used once, more than once, or not at all.
1. The laser with a depth of penetration of 0.3 mm
2. The laser type used to give a 'targeting beam'
3. The laser used in dermatological conditions of the face

9.

You are required to perform rigid bronchoscopy in an adult who has inhaled a peanut. The scrub nurse is having some difficulty assembling the instruments.

Correctly identify the following parts of the bronchoscope. Each response may be used once, more than once, or not at all.

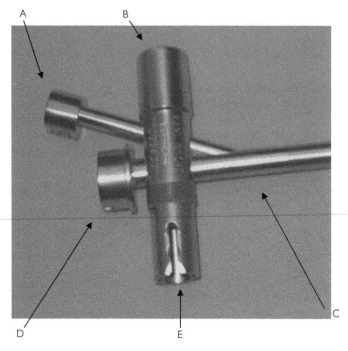

1. Connection to anaesthetic tubing
2. Suction port
3. Connection to light source

10. **Branches of the external carotid artery**
    A. Ascending pharyngeal
    B. Superior thyroid
    C. Lingual
    D. Facial
    E. Occipital
    F. Posterior auricular
    G. Superficial temporal
    H. Maxillary

    For each of the following statements, select the correct artery from the list above. Each response may be used once, more than once, or not at all.
    1. Winds around the body of the mandible
    2. Passes through the pterygopalatine fossa
    3. Is the dominant blood supply to a pharyngeal pouch
    4. Is the origin of the superior labial artery
    5. Is routinely ligated as part of a laryngectomy

11.
    A. Polymyositis
    B. Scleroderma
    C. Achalasia
    D. Ganglionic degeneration
    E. Carcinoma
    F. Pharyngeal pouch
    G. Barrett's oesophagus

    For each of the following situations, select the most likely diagnosis from the list above. Each response may be used once, more than once, or not at all.
    1. Chagas disease
    2. Aperistalsis, oesophageal dilatation, and failure of relaxation of the lower oesophageal sphincter
    3. Irregular appearance on contrast swallow
    4. May be associated with Raynaud's phenomenon

12.

    A. Pseudostratified ciliated columnar epithelium

    B. Stratified squamous epithelium

    C. Keratinized squamous epithelium

    D. Pavement epithelium without cilia

    E. Pseudostratified ciliated columnar epithelium with goblet cells

    F. Pseudostratified non-keratinized stratified squamous epithelium

Match each of the following anatomical locations with its correct epithelial type from the list above. Each response may be used once, more than once, or not at all.

    1. True vocal cords

    2. False cords

    3. Mastoid antrum

    4. Skin of pinna

    5. Trachea

13.

    A. Pemphigus

    B. Pemphigoid

    C. Candida

    D. Leucoplakia

    E. Erythroplakia

    F. Lichen planus

    G. Stevens–Johnson syndrome

    H. Behçet's disease

Which of the above-listed conditions is described in the following statements? Each response may be used once, more than once, or not at all.

    1. A high propensity to undergo malignant degeneration

    2. An idiosyncratic drug reaction

    3. Seen in conjunction with arthritis, eye pain, and genital ulcers

    4. Due to IgG autoantibodies targeted against desmosomal components

    5. Associated with skin 'target lesions'

1.

   1. A

Chronic lymphocytic thyroiditis is an autoimmune disease, associated with SLE, rheumatoid arthritis, pernicious anaemia, diabetes, and Sjögren syndrome. In 20% of cases, patients present with hypothyroidism. A rare association is thyroid lymphoma, usually B-cell non-Hodgkin's type and limited to the thyroid.

   2. H

This occurs often in postpartum patients, with acute symptoms of hyperthyroidism. It is associated with a family history of autoimmune thyroid disease. Fifty per cent present with a painless goitre. Radioactive iodine uptake is low in the initial hyperthyroid state. Management is with beta-blocking agents.

   3. G

This is usually viral in origin. The disease course commences with thyrotoxicosis, followed by euthyroid state, and then hypothyroidism, which can occasionally be permanent. Non-steroidal anti-inflammatory agents, beta blockers, and occasionally steroids are used to manage the condition.

Slatosky J, Shipton B, Wahba H. Thyroiditis: differential diagnosis and management. *American Family Physician* 2000;61:1047–1052.

2.

   1. J
   2. I
   3. G
   4. B
   5. C
   6. H

Proliferative verrucous leucoplasia is often associated with multiple lesions within the oral cavity, which progress to rough, raised areas. It is strongly associated with conversion to squamous cell carcinoma, including the verrucous variant. It often reoccurs.

Denture stomatitis is described as a red area, under a denture plate. Its outline sharply follows that of the denture.

All areas of unexplained leucoplakia should have a biopsy to exclude malignant disease. Larger areas (>200 mm²), particularly those that are non-homogeneous, those on the tongue or floor of mouth, and those in older age or female patients are at higher risk of malignant disease.

Erythroplakia usually suggests a more sinister pathology than leucoplakia, almost always showing dysplasia or carcinoma on a biopsy.

Chronic hyperplastic candidosis—proliferative areas adjacent to the denture. Can mimic malignancy. Requires a biopsy to exclude dysplasia. Patients should be counselled in good denture hygiene and to remove their plates overnight.

Chi AC, Day TA, Neville BW. Oral cavity and oropharyngeal squamous cell carcinoma—an update. *CA: A Cancer Journal for Clinicians* 2015;65:401–421.

3.

1. J

This represents a salivary duct carcinoma, an aggressive tumour, sometimes found with carcinoma ex pleomorphic. It is more common in older men. The clinical course is associated with early distant metastases, often of the lung, bone, liver, brain, and skin.

2. F

Mucoepidermoid carcinoma is the commonest salivary gland tumour. It is more common in females. It is divided into low and high grade by the number of mucin-containing cells in the specimen relative to the epidermoid cells. A large amount of mucin-producing cells indicates a low grade.

3. C

This pattern describes cribriform adenoid cystic carcinoma. There are three variants: tubular, cribriform, and solid. The solid subtype has the worst prognosis. Adenoid cystic carcinoma is often associated with perineural invasion.

International Agency for Research on Cancer. Tumours of the salivary glands. In: *WHO Classification of Head and Neck Tumours* (World Health Organization Classification of Tumours). 2017. Available at: https://www.iarc.fr/en/publications/pdfs-online/pat-gen/bb9/bb9-chap5.pdf.

4.

1. G

The accessory nerve (or spinal accessory nerve) is the 11th cranial nerve. It leaves the cranium through the jugular foramen along with the glossopharyngeal nerve (IX) and vagus nerve (X). There are two parts to the nerve. The spinal accessory nerve originates from neuronal cell bodies located in the cervical spinal cord and caudal medulla. Most are located in the spinal cord and ascend through the foramen magnum and exit the cranium through the jugular foramen. They are motor in function and innervate the sternocleidomastoid and trapezius muscles. The cranial root of the accessory nerve originates from cells located in the caudal medulla. They are found in the nucleus ambiguus and leave the brainstem with the fibres of the vagus nerve. They join the spinal root to exit the jugular foramen. They rejoin the vagus nerve and are distributed with the vagus nerve.

2. A

The lesser petrosal nerve carries preganglionic parasympathetic fibres from the inferior salivary nucleus via the otic ganglion to innervate the parotid gland. It is derived from the facial and glossopharyngeal nerve via the tympanic plexus and passes through the foramen ovale to synapse in the otic ganglion. Postsynaptic fibres leave the otic ganglion, join the auriculotemporal nerve, and innervate the parotid gland.

3. J

The chorda tympani, a branch of the facial nerve, carries special sensory fibres providing taste sensation from the anterior two-thirds of the tongue and presynaptic parasympathetic fibres to the submandibular ganglion, providing secretomotor innervation to two salivary glands: the submandibular gland and sublingual gland. The chorda tympani branches from the facial nerve, crosses the tympanic membrane, and exits through the petrotympanic fissure into the infratemporal fossa. It then joins the lingual nerve (V3) and supplies preganglionic parasympathetic fibres to the submandibular and sublingual salivary glands via the submandibular ganglion. Special sensory (taste) fibres from the chorda tympani supply the anterior two-thirds of the tongue via the lingual nerve.

5.

    1. A

    2. G

The sternocleidomastoid receives a segmental blood supply from the occipital artery, superior thyroid artery, and the transverse cervical artery.

    3. D

Poland syndrome consists of unilateral absence or hypoplasia of the pectoralis muscle, most frequently involving the sternocostal portion of the pectoralis major muscle, and a variable degree of ipsilateral hand and digit anomalies, including symbrachydactyly.

6.

    1. C or A

The greater superficial petrosal nerve passes through the Vidian canal to supply parasympathetic fibres to the glands of the nose and eye.

    2. F

The descendens hypoglossi is joined by the descendens cervicalis to form the ansa cervicalis.

    3. G

The lesser petrosal nerve (continuation of Jacobsen's nerve) is a branch of the glossopharyngeal nerve and transmits parasympathetic fibres to the parotid gland.

    4. G

    5. G

7.

    1. and 4. D

Adenoid cystic carcinoma is the most common malignancy of the submandibular, sublingual, and minor salivary glands. It exhibits perineural spread, and is associated with slow-growing distant metastases, particularly to the lungs.

    2. B

This is a classical history for a carcinoma arising in a pre-existing pleomorphic adenoma.

    3. F

Squamous cell carcinoma is the most likely diagnosis here.

8.

    1. B

    2. F

    3. C

The pulsed dye laser has been used in the treatment of skin lesions and more recently in certain conditions of the vocal cords

9.

    1. B

    2. A

    3. E

C represents the main lumen of the bronchoscope, and D is the port for introduction of the instruments.

10.

    1. D

    2. H

    3. A

    4. D

    5. B

11.

    1. D

Chagas disease is a parasitic disease caused by *Trypanosoma cruzi*, transmitted by blood-sucking insect vectors (reduviid bugs). Parasympathetic intramural denervation lesions can be dispersed irregularly, leading to dilated oesophagus (mega-oesophagus) or dilated and elongated (dolichol-mega-oesophagus).

    2. C

Patients with achalasia lack noradrenergic, noncholinergic inhibitory ganglion cells, leading to a hypertensive non-relaxed lower oesophageal sphincter.

    3. E

    4. B

Scleroderma may be seen as part of the CREST syndrome: Calcinosis; Raynaud's; (o)Esophageal dysmotility; Scleroderma; Telangiectasia.

12.

    1. F

    2. F

    3. D

    4. C

    5. E

13.

    1. E

Both erythroplakia and leucoplakia are pre-malignant, but the former is much more likely to undergo malignant change.

    2. G

Stevens–Johnson syndrome, which is the severe form of erythema multiforme, may be triggered by drugs (especially Septrin), viral infection, or food sensitivity. It is associated with characteristic 'target' lesions on the skin, most often on the hands.

3. H

Behçet's disease is a disease of unknown aetiology causing ulcers on the mucus membranes and skin.

4. A

Pemphigoid is due to IgG autoantibodies against basement membrane; it more often affects the elderly.

Pemphigus is due to IgG autoantibodies against desmosomal components; it more often affects the young, and commonly affects the oral mucosa.

5. G

1. Drug doses for children

A. 20 mL/kg
B. 10 mg/kg
C. 15 mg/kg
D. 0.1 mg/kg
E. 10 mcg/kg
F. 100 mcg/kg

Match each of the following drugs with its paediatric dose from the list above:
1. Paracetamol
2. Ibuprofen
3. Morphine sulphate
4. Intravenous/intraosseous dose of adrenaline in a cardiac arrest
5. Fluid challenge in severe dehydration

2. Investigation of paediatric hearing loss

A. Automated otoacoustic emission (OAE)
B. OAE + auditory brainstem response (ABR)
C. ABR
D. Visual reinforcement audiometry (VRA)
E. Pure tone audiometry (PTA)
F. Magnetic resonance imaging (MRI)
G. Computed tomography (CT)

What is the most appropriate first-line investigation from the above list for the following patients?
1. A neonate who spent 4 days in the neonatal intensive care unit (NICU) after birth for treatment of neonatal sepsis
2. A 5-year-old child with progressive bilateral sensorineural hearing loss
3. A non-syndromic child who failed their first OAE as part of the NHSP
4. A 3 year old child noted to have speech delay
5. A child with developmental delay unable to cooperate with subjective testing

3. **Branchial arch derivatives**
   A. Third branchial arch
   B. Second branchial arch
   C First branchial cleft
   D. Third branchial pouch
   E. Fourth branchial arch

   Based on the embryology of the developing fetus, choose the origin of the following structures from the list above:
   1. Stylopharyngeus
   2. Muscles of facial expression
   3. External auditory canal
   4. Inferior parathyroids
   5. Thyroid cartilage

4. **Craniosynostosis**
   A. Lamboid suture
   B. Metopic suture
   C. Coronal suture
   D. Sagittal suture

   Match each of the following suture lines to their position on the cranial vault listed above:
   1. Separates the frontal bones from the parietal bones
   2. Separates the frontal bones
   3. Separates the occipital bone from the two parietal bones
   4. Separates the two parietal bones

5. **Paediatric infections**
   A. Non-tuberculous mycobacteria
   B. Congenital toxoplasmosis
   C. Congenital rubella
   D. Hand, foot, and mouth
   E. Kawasaki disease
   F. Measles
   G. Chicken pox

   Match the following descriptions to the likely causative infection from the list above:
   1. Strawberry tongue, desquamating rash, red blistering lips
   2. Chorioretinitis, hydrocephalus, intracerebral calcification
   3. Painless lymph node mass with a violaceous hue
   4. Jaundice, intrauterine growth restriction, sensorineural hearing loss, congenital heart defects
   5. Pyrexial, mouth ulcers, maculopapular or vesicular rash on palms

6.

    A. 4 joules/kg
    B. 0.1 mg/kg
    C. (Age/4) + 4
    D. (Age in years + 4) × 2
    E. (Age in months/2) + 4
    F. 20 mL/kg

The 'WETFLAG' acronym is used for calculations during paediatric advanced life support scenarios. How are the following calculated?
1. Weight for a child older than 1 year
2. Energy
3 Endotracheal tube size
4. Lorazepam
5. Adrenaline 1:10,000

7.

    A. Cytomegalovirus
    B. Rubella
    C. Mumps
    D. Parvovirus
    E. Measles
    F. Toxoplasmosis
    G. *Treponema pallidum*
    H. Norwalk virus
    I. Varicella zoster
    J. Herpes simplex

For each of the following questions, select the most likely infection from the list above. Each response may be used once, more than once, or not at all.
1. Which infection is the commonest cause of infective congenital sensorineural hearing loss?
2. Which infection is most commonly associated with unilateral sensorineural hearing loss acquired in childhood?
3. Which infection has been implicated in the aetiology of otosclerosis?

8.

A. Apert syndrome

B. Alport syndrome

C. Crouzon syndrome

D. Treacher Collins syndrome

E. Pfeiffer syndrome

F. Saethre–Chotzen syndrome

G. Jackson–Weiss syndrome

For each of the following questions, select the most likely syndrome from the list above. Each response may be used once, more than once, or not at all.

1. Which syndrome exhibits autosomal dominant inheritance and often results in brachycephaly, midfacial hypoplasia, and normal intelligence?

2. Which syndrome exhibits autosomal dominant inheritance and often results in auricular malformations, conductive hearing loss, and normal intelligence?

3. Which syndrome is associated in males with progressive sensorineural hearing loss, haematuria, and chronic renal failure?

9.

A. Fibroblast growth factor receptor 1

B. Fibroblast growth factor receptor 2

C. Fibroblast growth factor receptor 3

D. Fibroblast growth factor receptor 4

E. Collagen type 1

F. Collagen type 2

G. Collagen type 3

H. Collagen type 4

Select the correct responses for the following questions from the list above. Each response may be used once, more than once, or not at all.

1. Achondroplasia is associated with a mutation in which gene?

2. Crouzon syndrome is associated with a mutation in which gene?

3. Apert syndrome is associated with a mutation in which gene?

10.

A. Acromegaly
B. Acrocephaly
C. Brachycephaly
D. Colpocephaly
E. Lissencephaly
F. Microcephaly
G. Plagiocephaly
H. Scaphocephaly
I. Trigonocephaly

Select the correct response from the list above for the following questions. Each response may be used once, more than once, or not at all.

1. Premature fusion of the coronal suture results in which abnormality?
2. What is the most common craniofacial abnormality found in Apert syndrome?
3. Which craniofacial abnormality is most common?

11. A 5-year-old boy presents to the Accident and Emergency department with noisy breathing

A. Flexible nasendoscopy
B. Immediate tracheostomy
C. Laryngoscopy and intubation in the operating theatre
D. Examination of the mouth
E. Chest X-ray
F. Soft tissue X-ray of the neck
G. Rigid bronchoscopy
H. CT scan of the neck

To obtain a diagnosis, which management would be most appropriate in the following situations? Each response may be used once, more than once, or not at all.

1. The child is febrile, tachycardic, drooling and has marked odynophagia
2. The child may have inhaled a foreign body
3. The child has been stridulous for many months
4. The child was diagnosed with tonsillitis 2 days ago

12. **A child is found, at his neonatal screening test, to have a severe sensorineural hearing loss**
    A. Pendred syndrome
    B. Usher syndrome
    C. Waardenburg syndrome
    D. Alport syndrome
    E. Branchio-oto-renal syndrome
    F. Neurofibromatosis type II
    G. Jervell–Lange-Nielsen syndrome
    H. Treacher Collins syndrome
    I. Stickler syndrome

    Which of the syndromes listed above would most likely apply in the following situations? Each response may be used once, more than once, or not at all.
    1. The child has widely spaced eyes
    2. The child has Hirschsprung's disease
    3. The child has retinal flecks
    4. The child has a goitre
    5. The child as a prolonged QT interval on the electrocardiogram (ECG)

13.
    A. Autosomal dominant
    B. Autosomal recessive
    C. X-linked
    D. Usually sporadic
    E. Variable penetrance
    F. Imprinting
    G. Variable expressivity

    For each of the following conditions, select the most appropriate description from the list above. Each response may be used once, more than once, or not at all.
    1. Waardenburg syndrome
    2. Alport syndrome
    3. Usher syndrome
    4. Apert syndrome
    5. van der Woude syndrome

14.

    A. Polysomnogram

    B. Overnight oxygen saturation monitoring

    C. Proceed direct to adenotonsillectomy

    D. Genetic screening

    E. X-ray of postnasal space

    F. Sleep nasendoscopy

For each of the following clinical situations, select the most appropriate management of the patient from the list above. Each response may be used once, more than once, or not at all.

1. In clear-cut cases of obstructive sleep apnoea in a child of 5 years
2. When central apnoea is suspected
3. When obstructive sleep apnoea may be suspected in a child, but the clinical situation suggests that this may not be the case (e.g. if the child has small tonsils, and/or if the child is breathing freely through the nose)

1.

  1. C
  2. B
  3. D
  4. E
  5. A

2.

  1. B
  2. E
  3. A
  4. D
  5. C

The newborn hearing screening programme consists of two pathways. One for the well baby and another for babies who have spent 48 hours or more in a NICU. Babies with other medical problems that put them at risk of hearing loss (e.g. meningitis) are referred directly to audiology for screening. Visual reinforcement audiometry is the subjective test of choice for developmentally normal children over the age of 6 months up to 2–3 years

3.

  1. A
  2. B
  3. C
  4. D
  5. E.

The branchial apparatus develops between the second to sixth intrauterine week. Each arch contains an artery, nerve, muscles, and cartilage. Clefts are ectoderm lined and separate the arches externally, while pouches are endoderm lined separating the arches internally.

4.

  1. C
  2. B
  3. A
  4. D

5.

1. E
2. B
3. A
4. C
5. D

Congenital rubella is normally seen in neonates infected/exposed during the first trimester of pregnancy. The classic triad of symptoms consists of sensorineural deafness, congenital heart disease, and eye defects. Kawasaki disease is an acute vasculitic disease of childhood. Although most patients recover with little long-lasting effect, coronary artery aneurysm may occur in up to 25% of those untreated hence aspirin and immunoglobulin therapy is initiated.

6.

1. D
2. A
3. C
4. B
5. B

The WETFLAG algorithm is used in paediatric emergency scenarios and is used to calculate the following:

W Weight: Up to 1 year: (age in months/2) + 4
   More than 1 year: (age in years + 4) × 2
E Electricity: 4 joules/kg/biphasic
T Endotracheal tube: Internal diameter (age/4 + 4) = --- mm
   Length: Oropharyngeal tube (age /2 +12) = -- cm
   Nasopharyngeal tube (age /2+ 15) = --- cm
F Fluids: Medical/cardiac arrest: 20 mL/kg
   Trauma cases: initial bolus 10 mL/kg, then second 10 mL/kg
L Lorazepam: 0.1 mg/kg intravenous/intraosseous
A Adrenaline: 0.1 mL/kg of 1:10,000 = 10 mcg/kg
G Glucose: 2 mL/kg of 10% dextrose

7.

1. A

Cytomegalovirus is the commonest cause of congenital hearing loss.

2. C

Hearing loss from mumps is acquired in childhood. It tends to occur after an episode of parotitis and is usually unilateral and may be profound.

3. E

Measles virus has been associated with otosclerotic foci and remains a possible aetiological factor in the development of the disease.

8.

1. C

Crouzon syndrome is inherited in an autosomal dominant pattern and results in abnormalities of skull due to premature fusion of cranial sutures. The coronal and sagittal sutures most commonly involved. Other associated features include midface hypoplasia, exorbitism, glue ear, a high-arched palate, and normal intelligence.

2. D

Treacher Collins syndrome exhibits autosomal dominant inheritance with complete penetrance and variable expression, up to 60% of cases are spontaneous new mutations. Features of the condition include maxillary hypoplasia, down sloping palpebral fissures and 'parrot face' appearance. Patients frequently have microtia or atresia with a predominantly conductive hearing loss. Most patients have normal intelligence.

3. B

This condition is inherited in an X-linked or autosomal dominant fashion is associated with progressive sensorineural hearing loss, nephritis, haematuria and chronic renal failure.

9.

1. C
2. B
3. B

10.

1. C
2. C

Bicoronal synostosis resulting in brachycephaly is the suture fusion found most often in Apert and Crouzon syndromes.

3. H

Premature fusion of the sagittal suture is the most common, resulting in scaphocephaly.

The frequency of occurrence of the various types of craniosynostosis in the population is approximately as follows:

- Sagittal 50–58%
- Coronal 20–29%
- Metopic 4–10%
- Lambdoid 2–4%.

11.

1. C

This symptom complex suggests epiglottitis, and the child should be transferred immediately to theatre for intubation.

2. G

The most reliable way of making a diagnosis in this situation is to perform rigid bronchoscopy.

3. A

Flexible nasendoscopy is likely to suggest a diagnosis in this instance; he/she may have laryngeal papillomatosis or a laryngeal haemangioma.

4. D

A simple examination of the tonsils with a tongue depressor will confirm the diagnosis.

12.

1. C

Along with abnormal pigmentation of iris, hair, and skin, Waardenburg syndrome is associated with dystopia canthorum (widely spaced medial canthi) and Hirschsprung disease.

2. C

3. D

Alport syndrome is associated with progressive renal failure and retinal flecks.

4. A

Pendred syndrome is associated with goitre (usually evident before puberty) that results in hypothyroidism in 50% of cases and euthyroidism in the other half.

5. G

The prolonged QT interval in the ECG of patients with Jervell–Lange-Nielsen syndrome results in syncopal attacks or death.

13.

1. A

2. C

3. B

4. A

5. A or E

14.

1. C

No investigation is required and if the clinical history is strong enough, the child may be placed on the waiting list for adenotonsillectomy.

2. A

A polysomnogram is useful when central apnoea is suspected: in this case, there will be no respiratory effort when the saturations fall, and this will be detected by the movement sensors on the chest wall.

3. B

Overnight saturation monitoring may be useful if there is any doubt as to whether the child genuinely has OSA.

1.

A. Nodular
B. Pigmented
C. Superficial
D. Morpheaform/sclerosing
E. Lentigo maligna
F. Actinic keratosis
G. Amelanotic

Which form of basal cell carcinoma (BCC) from the list above is most common in the following scenarios?
1. Most common, raised hard skin, pearly edge, superficial telangiectasia
2. Raised hard skin, pearly edge, darkened colour
3. Rarest form, can resemble psoriasis or eczema
4. Resembles a scar, most difficult to treat as more likely to have involved margins

2.

A. Granulomatosis with polyangiitis (GPA)
B. GPA with eosinophilia
C. Tuberculosis
D. Syphilis
E. Sarcoidosis
F. Iatrogenic septal perforation
G. Rhinosporidiosis
H. Rhinoscleroma

In each of the following situations, give the most appropriate cause from the list above for nasal crusting:

1. A patient has had previous septal surgery and notices whistling when breathing through the nose
2. A patient has lung infiltrates/nodules on chest X-ray. The general practitioner has been concerned regarding the kidney function. The cytoplasmic antineutrophil cytoplasmic antibody (cANCA) assay is positive
3. A patient has bilateral hilar lymphadenopathy on chest X-ray and has red to purple indurated plaques affecting the skin of the nose and cheeks
4. A male patient from Sri Lanka presents with nasal crusting, and lesions in the oropharynx and external genitalia
5. A male patient from Egypt presents with an infection caused by *Klebsiella rhinoscleromatis*

3.

A. Foreign body
B. Pyogenic granuloma
C. Osler–Weber–Rendu syndrome
D. Traumatic
E. Sinonasal malignancy
F. Mucosal melanoma
G. Inverted papilloma

From the list above, give the most likely cause of epistaxis in each of the following situations:

1. A 2-year-old boy presents with unilateral, foul-smelling nasal discharge and occasional nose bleeds
2. A pregnant lady presents with a red swelling on the nasal septum which bleeds easily with contact
3. A male patient presents with a history of epistaxis; on further examination he has telangiectasia around the lips. He is being investigated for gastrointestinal bleeding

4.

    A. Pyogenic granuloma
    B. Rhabdomyosarcoma
    C. Squamous cell carcinoma
    D. Adenocarcinoma
    E. Inverted papilloma
    F. Juvenile angiofibroma
    G. Mucosal melanoma

Which of the nasal masses in the list above is most likely in each of the following clinical situations?

1. A carpenter presents with a 1-month history of blood-stained nasal discharge, unilateral nasal obstruction, and a numb face
2. A 67-year-old gentleman who has worked in the textile industry presents with a numb face, nasal obstruction, and bloody nasal discharge
3. A 16-year-old boy presents with nasal obstruction and recurrent episodes of epistaxis which are getting more severe
4. A 2-year-old boy presents with bloody nasal discharge, computed tomography (CT) scanning reveals a soft tissue mass within the maxillary sinus eroding bone
5. A 32-year-old pregnant lady presents with a lesion on Little's area of the septum which bleeds easily

5.

    A. T3, N1
    B. T3, N0, M0
    C. T4a
    D. T1, N2A
    E. T2
    F. T4b
    G. T3
    H. T4, N3

From the list above, apply the correct staging for the following sinonasal malignancies:

1. A patient presents with an adenocarcinoma originating from the ethmoid sinus extending into the medial wall of the orbit and the cribriform plate. There are no regional nodes or distant metastasis on radiological imaging
2. A patient presents with a mucosal melanoma affecting the mucosa of the middle turbinate. There are pathological nodes in level II
3. A patient presents with a maxillary sinus tumour extending onto the skin of the nose and cheek
4. A patient presents with nasopharyngeal carcinoma extending to involve the parapharyngeal space
5. A patient presents with a history of nasal obstruction and facial numbness. CT scanning demonstrates a malignant tumour of the maxillary sinus involving the posterior wall

6.

A. Basal cell carcinoma
B. Squamous cell carcinoma
C. Bowen's disease
D. Lupus pernio
E. Malignant melanoma
F. Actinic keratosis

From the histological diagnoses listed above, which is the most likely in each of the following situations?

1. An elderly man presents with a patch of thick, crusting skin on the scalp. Biopsy demonstrates atypical keratinocyte proliferation
2. A 32-year-old lady presents with purple indurated plaques on the cheeks. Her serum angiotensin-converting enzyme (ACE) is raised
3. An elderly lady presents with a well-demarcated red plaque on the right temple. Histology confirms abnormal squamous cells throughout the epidermis but not invading the dermis
4. An elderly lady presents with a red plaque on the temple. Histology confirms abnormal squamous cells within the epidermis and invading the dermis
5. A 55-year-old female patient presents with a waxy scar-like plaque just below the left eye. Biopsy confirms malignancy

7.   Aesthetic facial analysis

A. Trichion
B. Glabella
C. Nasion
D. Radix
E. Sellion
F. Rhinion
G. Supratip
H. Tip
I. Subnasale
J. Superior sulcus
K. Labrale superius
L. Stomion
M. Labrale inferius
N. Mentolabial sulcus
O. Pogonion
P. Menton

For each of the following statements, identify the structure described from the list above:

1. It is the point cephalic to the tip
2. It is the junction of the bony and cartilaginous nasal dorsum
3. It is the soft tissue correlate of the deepest point of the forehead at the nasal root (nasion)
4. It is the most inferior point on the chin
5. It is the most prominent projection of frontal bone just above the nasofrontal suture
6. It is the junction of the columella and the cutaneous upper lip
7. It is the mucocutaneous junction of the lower lip

8.

  A. Type I
  B. Type II
  C. Type III
  D. Type IV

In the Gell and Coombs classification of hypersensitivity reactions (listed above), match the correct description in each of the following cases:

1. It is IgG mediated with a mechanism of antibody directed against a cell surface antigen leading to cell destruction through complement activation
2. It is a cell-mediated delayed hypersensitivity reaction. Mechanism is T-helper 1 cells activate macrophages or CD 8 cells giving cellular damage and inflammation. This type of hypersensitivity is associated with granulomatous diseases
3. It is an immediate IgE-mediated reaction. The mechanism involves the degranulation of mast cells
4. Is an immune complex-mediated IgG hypersensitivity reaction. The mechanism involves the deposition of antigen–antibody deposition on the surfaces of small vasculature and kidney glomeruli. Is a cause of post-streptococcal glomerulonephritis

9.   Systemic infectious and inflammatory diseases

  A. Heerfordt syndrome
  B. Cogan syndrome
  C. Relapsing perichondritis
  D. Behçet syndrome
  E. Sjögren syndrome
  F. Pemphigus vulgaris
  G. Pemphigoid
  H. Human immunodeficiency virus
  I. Granulomatosis with polyangiitis (GPA, formerly known as Wegner's granulomatosis)
  J. GPA with eosinophilia (formerly known as Churg–Strauss syndrome)
  K. Amyloidosis
  L. Leprosy (Hansen's disease)

Match each of the following situations with the disease listed above which best fits the symptoms and signs:

1. A young gentleman presents with painful bleeding oral ulcerations. This disease is characterized by loosening of the epidermal–dermal junction. Antibodies to desmoglein are present. A positive Nikolsky sign is present
2. A young woman presents with a relapsing and remitting autoimmune disorder. She has oral and genital ulcerations along with iritis and a progressive sensorineural hearing loss
3. A 50-year-old male following a fever presents with parotitis, uveitis, and a facial nerve palsy
4. A 34-year-old female has been seen in the general ENT clinic with a bilateral progressive hearing loss and uveitis
5. A 52-year-old female has presented to the local ENT department with auricular chondritis on two occasions; she has recently been found to have a 'sabre-toothed' trachea
6. A 54-year-old African male presents with painless and insensate skin patches along with ulceration and perforation of the nasal septum

10. Nasal cavity and paranasal sinus tumours

A. Olfactory neuroblastoma (esthesioneuroblastoma)

B. Chondrosarcoma

C. Adenocarcinoma

D. Rhabdomyosarcoma

E. Adenoid cystic

F. Squamous cell carcinoma

G. Inverted papilloma

H. Adenocarcinoma

I. Mucoepidermoid carcinoma

From the list above, choose the most appropriate diagnosis in each of the following situations:

1. It is associated with exposure to wood dust and lacquers
2. A 12-year-old presents with epistaxis and is found on examination to have a pale, gelatinous grape structure in the right nasal vestibule
3. Most common salivary gland tumour of the nose and postnasal space
4. A midline tumour affecting older patients demonstrating matrix calcification and endosteal cortical scalloping on CT scanning
5. Has a characteristic 'dumb-bell' mass extending across the cribriform plate on imaging and is found to have a 'small round blue cell' appearance on histology after staining

11. Causes of anosmia

A. Kallman syndrome

B. Foster Kennedy syndrome

C. Alzheimer's disease

D. Chronic rhinosinusitis

E. Fungal sinus disease

F. Foreign body

G. Trauma

H. Iatrogenic

I. Schizophrenia

From the list above, which is the most likely aetiology of anosmia in each of the following situations?

1. A 14-year-old girl presents with anosmia; on further questioning it is noted she is being investigated by her general practitioner for not entering puberty
2. A 75-year-old gentleman presents with anosmia, and is also noted to have personality changes with unusually aggressive behaviour and loss of memory
3. A 35-year-old man presents with anosmia, headaches, and loss of vision. On examination, papilloedema is found
4. A 25-year-old gentleman complains of hearing voices. His family state that he is becoming socially withdrawn

12. Causes of a septal perforation

A. Granulomatosis with polyangiitis (GPA)
B. Iatrogenic
C. Trauma
D. GPA with eosinophilia
E. Sarcoidosis
F. Tuberculosis
G. Relapsing perichondritis
H. Syphilis
I. Cocaine abuse
J. Leprosy
K. Carcinoma
L. T-cell type non-Hodgkin lymphoma (lethal midline granuloma)

From the list above, select the most likely cause of a septal perforation in each of the following situations:

1. A 50-year-old gentleman presents with a septal perforation; he has a high serum cANCA and lung nodules on chest X-ray
2. A 26-year-old gentleman presents with a septal perforation, having suffered a myocardial infarction 1 year ago; he exhibits antisocial behaviour
3. A 50-year-old gentleman presents with a nasal septal perforation, bilateral hilar lymphadenopathy on chest X-ray, and a high serum calcium
4. A 56-year-old Asian male presents with ulcerative septal perforation, foul-smelling mucopurulent and bloody nasal discharge, facial swelling, and recurrent fevers

13.

A. Suprabullar recess
B. Hiatus semilunaris
C. Agger nasi cell
D. Bulla ethmoidalis
E. Kuhn cell
F. Haller cell
G. Uncinate process
H. Frontal process of the maxilla
I. Middle meatus
J. Inferior meatus
K. Superior meatus
L. Supreme meatus
M. Sphenoethmoidal cell (Onodi)

Select the correct anatomical structure from the list above based on the following descriptions. Each response may be used once, more than once, or not at all.

1. Two-dimensional space lying between the bulla and the uncinate process
2. Anterior wall of the frontal recess
3. Embryologically derived from the second basal lamella

14.

A. Lower lateral cartilage
B. Upper lateral cartilage
C. Nasal bones
D. Septal cartilage
E. Vomer
F. Perpendicular plate of ethmoid

For each of the following questions, select the correct answer from the list above. Each response may be used once, more than once, or not at all.

1. In order to achieve upward tip rotation in rhinoplasty surgery, which structure may be trimmed cephalically?

2. Which structure contributes most to columella show?

3. Which structure is most likely to be damaged during the incisions in an open rhinoplasty?

1.

    1. A
    2. B
    3. C
    4. D

2.

    1. F
    2. A
    3. E
    4. G
    5. H

Septal perforations cause nasal crusting and frequent epistaxis, smaller perforations classically whistle on nasal breathing. GPA (formerly known as Wegner's granulomatosis) is a vascular disease affecting small- and medium-sized vessels. The inflammation classically affects the nose, lungs, and kidneys, although it may affect any other organ system. The classical chest X-ray for GPA demonstrates lung infiltrates or nodules, compared to sarcoidosis in which the chest X-ray typically demonstrates bilateral hilar lymphadenopathy. The blood test for GPA is cANCA, the antigen being the enzyme proteinase 3 (PR3). This compares to GPA with eosinophilia (formerly known as Churg–Strauss syndrome) for which the blood test is perinuclear ANCA and the antigen is myeloperoxidase (MPO). GPA with eosinophilia is also a vascular disease affecting small- and medium-sized vessels. The classical presentation is in three stages: first, an allergic phase including asthma and signs and symptoms suggesting chronic rhinosinusitis. The second phase is the eosinophilia in which there is a high level of these types of white cells in the blood and tissues; this phase is usually associated with malaise, fever, and night sweats. The third phase is the vasculitis. Rhinosporidiosis is caused by a protist, classified under Mesomycetozoea. It is a disease endemic to South India, Sri Lanka, South America, and Africa. Within the nasal cavity, the floor of the nose, inferior turbinate, and nasopharynx are typically affected. The oropharynx, conjunctiva, and external genitalia are other common sites affected. Within the nasal cavity, pink/red polyps can be found which have a 'strawberry' appearance and bleed easily. Symptoms include nasal obstruction, rhinorrhoea, cough, wheezing, and conjunctivitis. Rhinoscleroma is a chronic granulomatous disease caused by *Klebsiella rhinoscleromatis*. The disease has three stages, the first being the catarrhal/strophic stage which mimics a rhinitis picture progressing to nasal crusting. The second is the granulomatous stage in which the nasal mucosa becomes a bluish-red colour. Nasal bleeding and deformity occur in this stage. The third stage is the sclerotic stage. Apart from the nose, the upper respiratory tract can be involved which has a very bleak prognosis due to involvement of the larynx, trachea, and bronchi.

3.

1. A
2. B
3. C

Any child with unilateral nasal discharge must be suspected of having a foreign body lodged within the nasal cavity. Pyogenic granulomas are a form of capillary haemangioma. These lesions tend to occur on Little's area within the nose and are very friable. Classically, they enlarge with pregnancy and begin involuting sometime after with hormonal stabilization. Osler–Weber–Rendu syndrome (hereditary haemorrhagic telangiectasia) is an autosomal dominant condition associated with telangiectasia, recurrent epistaxis, and a positive family history. Lesions occur within the gastrointestinal tract, the lungs, and arteriovenous malformations within the brain. There is an association with migraine and epilepsy.

4.

1. D
2. C
3. F
4. B
5. A

Squamous cell carcinoma is still the most common sinonasal malignancy. It is associated with textile working and heavy metal exposure. Hardwood exposure is associated with sinonasal adenocarcinoma, which typically begins in the ethmoid sinus. Squamous cell carcinoma affects the maxillary sinus, nasal cavity, and then ethmoids, in order of frequency. Recurrent epistaxis in a teenage boy, especially symptoms which are severe and getting worse, is very suggestive of juvenile angiofibroma. For any head and neck malignancy in a child, rhabdomyosarcoma should be considered: squamous cell carcinoma and adenocarcinoma would be extremely unlikely in this scenario. Pyogenic granuloma is a benign capillary haemangioma which is associated with hormonal changes in pregnancy.

5.

1. B
2. A
3. C
4. E
5. G

It is important to recognize mucosal melanoma begins at a T3 stage due to its poorer prognosis than cutaneous melanoma. Lymph node involvement in melanoma is not staged in the same way as squamous cell carcinoma of the head and neck. Lymph nodes in melanoma are assessed as NX, meaning they cannot be assessed; N0, none are present; and N1, meaning there is regional lymph node involvement.

6.

1. F
2. D
3. C
4. B
5. A

The distinguishing feature of malignancy is the invasion of the dermis. Bowen's disease is effectively squamous cell carcinoma *in situ*. Once it has spread through the dermis (transgression of the basement membrane) it becomes frank malignancy, squamous cell carcinoma. Actinic keratosis (also termed solar keratosis) is usually found in elderly patients with ultraviolet (UV) light-damaged skin. The lesions have three main outcomes: they may regress, remain stable, or go on to become invasive disease. There is a low malignant transformation potential of a single lesion, but patients generally have many of these lesions, greater than half of squamous cell carcinoma lesions are thought to have arisen in lesions previously being diagnosed as actinic keratosis. Sclerosing or morpheaform basal cell carcinoma resembles a scar with a waxy appearance.

7.

1. G
2. F
3. D
4. P
5. B
6. I
7. M

8.

1. B
2. D
3. A
4. D

9.

1. F
2. D
3. A
4. B
5. C
6. L

Cogan syndrome is assumed to be autoimmune in aetiology, a non-syphilitic interstitial keratitis with vestibuloauditory symptoms similar to Ménière's disease. Relapsing perichondritis is an inflammatory disorder which causes episodic inflammation of cartilaginous structures; the most commonly affected structures are the auricular cartilages with approximately 50% developing airway involvement. Pemphigus vulgaris is an autoimmune condition affecting the skin and mucous membranes. Symptoms include painful oral ulcers, vesicles which rupture, laryngeal involvement, and epistaxis. The antibody is to desmoglein, a family of cadherins which are transmembrane proteins involved in cell adhesion. Desmoglein 3 is found in the oral and oropharyngeal mucosa and desmoglein 1 is found in the skin. In Nikolsky sign, the top layers of the skin slip away from the lower layers when slightly rubbed. This is a distinguishing sign from pemphigoid which is a group of autoimmune diseases, mainly IgG mediated, which can affect the skin. Pemphigoid may be either bullous or cicatricial (affecting the mucous membranes). Gestational pemphigoid is also described. In distinction to pemphigus, there is no acantholysis. Heerfordt syndrome—uveoparotid disease—is a variant of sarcoidosis; patients typically present with parotitis, uveitis, and facial nerve palsy.

10.

   1. C
   2. D
   3. E
   4. B
   5. A

Olfactory neuroblastoma (esthesioneuroblastoma) is a tumour originating from the olfactory epithelium, therefore most commonly arising from either the cribriform plate, upper septum, or the superior turbinate. On histology, olfactory neuroblastomas have a characteristic 'small round blue cell' appearance with staining. Certain sarcomas, mucosal melanoma, and non-Hodgkin's lymphoma among others have a similar characteristic appearance. The Kadish staging system is commonly used for these tumours with stage A being confined to the nasal cavity, stage B extending to the paranasal sinuses, and stage 3 extension beyond the paranasal sinuses. They are locally aggressive tumours, and 10–30% will have distant spread at presentation. Chondrosarcoma is a rare midline tumour. Histologically, they are typically graded I to III, well to poorly differentiated, with the differentiation depending on the chondroid to myxoid ratio. Differentiating a chondroma from a low-grade chondrosarcoma can be difficult: benign tumours are usually less than 3 cm in size, and anything larger than this would be suspicious for the sarcoma variant. Skull base lesions can be very difficult to manage and have a poorer prognosis due to the close proximity of critical neurovascular structures. There is a reported recurrence rate of up to 85% for these tumours. Rhabdomyosarcoma should be suspected in children and adolescents presenting with symptoms and signs suggestive of malignancy. In the areas of the body covered with mucous membranes, it classically has a botryoid (bunch of grapes) appearance.

11.

   1. A
   2. C
   3. B
   4. I

Kallman syndrome is a failure to start or complete puberty with an associated loss of smell. It may affect females and males, although is more commonly found in males. The gonadotropin-releasing hormone (GnRH)-expressing neurons originate in an area of the developing brain called the olfactory placode; they then pass through the cribriform plate then to the olfactory bulb, where the sense of smell is generated. From there they migrate into what will become the hypothalamus. Any problems with the development of the olfactory bulb will prevent the progression of the GnRH-expressing neurons through it. If the GnRH-expressing neurons are prevented from reaching the hypothalamus, no GnRH will be released, so in turn no follicle-stimulating hormone (FSH) or luteinizing hormone (LH) will be released which results in the failure of puberty and deficient production of testosterone in men, and oestrogen and progesterone in women. In Kallmann syndrome, the olfactory bulb is missing or not fully developed which gives rise to the additional symptom of lack of sense of smell (anosmia) or vastly reduced sense of smell (hyposmia). Foster Kennedy syndrome is unilateral anosmia, optic atrophy, and papilloedema secondary to a frontal lobe mass. Neurodegenerative disorders such as Alzheimer's and Parkinson's diseases must always be thought of in dealing with patients, especially elderly individuals as anosmia and hyposmia are early signs.

12.

1. A
2. I
3. E
4. L

Sarcoidosis is associated with a high serum ACE concentration and elevated serum calcium concentration. GPA is associated with a raised level of serum cANCA. The classical chest X-ray findings in sarcoidosis are bilateral hilar lymphadenopathy compared to nodules or infiltrates in GPA. Any young person having a septal perforation should be suspected of substance abuse, especially with a history of myocardial infarction which would be very unusual within this age group. Any substance abuse may be associated with psychological problems. T-cell type non-Hodgkin's lymphoma (lethal midline granuloma) is characterized by a progressive ulceration and necrosis of the nasal cavity involving other midline facial tissues. Treatment generally consists of radiotherapy for early-stage and chemoradiotherapy for later-stage disease although prognosis is very poor with a median survival of 6 months, and a 5-year survival rate of 20%.

13.

1. B
2. C
3. D

The hiatus semilunaris is a two dimensional space lying between the bulla and the uncinate process. It is the common drainage site of the maxillary antrum, and anterior ethmoid sinuses. The agger nasi cell is the most anterior pneumatized cell and is anterior to the vertical attachment of the middle turbinate. It forms the anterior boundary of the frontal recess.

14.

1. A
2. D
3. A

Cephalic trimming of the lower lateral cartilages will, with healing, cause the tip to rotate upwards. The lower lateral cartilages are very superficial and are easily damaged in the initial incisions in an open-approach rhinoplasty.

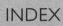

INDEX

Note: page numbers followed by *q* refer to questions, and those followed by *a* refer to answers.

For the benefit of digital users, indexed terms that span two pages (e.g., 52–53) may, on occasion, appear on only one of those pages.

A

Abbe flap 116q, 128–29a
accessory nerve *see* spinal accessory nerve
achalasia 23a, 177q, 182a
achondroplasia 188q, 194a
acinic cell carcinoma, in pregnancy 64q, 81a
acoustic neuroma
   clinical signs 161q, 168a
   imaging modality 159q, 167a
   middle cranial fossa approach 25q, 38a
actinic keratosis 200q, 206–7a
activated partial thromboplastin time (APTT) 149q, 156a
adenocarcinoma, sinonasal *see* sinonasal adenocarcinoma
adenoid cystic carcinoma
   clinical features 175q, 181a
   cribriform 173q, 180a
   nose and paranasal space 202q, 208a
adenotonsillectomy 104a
adrenaline
   anaphylaxis 79a
   bupivacaine with, maximum volume 147q, 154a
   lidocaine with, safe dose 13q, 23a, 147q, 154a
   paediatric dose 185q, 187q, 192a, 193a
advanced life support, paediatric 187q, 193a
aesthesioneuroblastoma *see* olfactory neuroblastoma
aesthetics
   facial analysis 113q, 121q, 127a, 134a, 200q, 207a
   nose 114q, 128a
ageing, facial 122q, 135a
agger nasi cell 203q, 209a
airflow resistance, narrowed trachea 90q, 101a
AJCC *see* American Joint Committee on Cancer
Alexander malformation 41a
allergic fungal sinusitis 125a
allergic response 118q, 129–30a
allergic rhinitis 8q, 20a
Alport syndrome 167a, 188q, 194a
   clinical presentation 158q, 165a
   hearing loss 44a, 190q, 195a
   inheritance 190q, 195a
Alzheimer disease 202q, 208a
American Joint Committee on Cancer (AJCC) staging

HPV-positive tonsillar carcinoma 69q, 84a
   see also tonsillar carcinoma
   melanoma 114q, 128a
   see also TNM classification
American Society of Anesthesiologists (ASA) grade 14q,
   23a, 24a
aminoglycosides, ototoxicity 32q, 42a
ammonia 110q, 126a, 135a
anaesthesia
   induction, child with history of choking 94q, 103a
   paediatric microlaryngoscopy and
      bronchoscopy 95q, 104a
analysis of variance 156a
anaphylactic shock 79a
angiofibroma, juvenile nasal *see* juvenile nasal angiofibroma
anosmia
   ammonia sensitivity 110q, 126a
   causes 135a, 202q, 208a
ansa cervicalis 174q, 181a
anterior ethmoidal nerve 21a
anterior lacrimal crest 108q, 125a
anterior lateral free flap 134a
antibiotics, mechanisms of action 12q, 22a, 142q, 151a
anticancer drugs, clinical trials 7q, 19a
anticoagulants
   indications for reversal 10q, 21a
   new oral 11q, 22a
   see also warfarin
antineutrophil cytoplasmic antibodies (ANCA) 126a,
   131–32a
antrochoanal polyp 120q, 133a
Apert syndrome 97q, 105a
   craniofacial abnormality 189q, 194a
   gene mutation 188q, 194a
   inheritance 190q, 195a
apixaban 22a
apnoea
   central 191q, 195a
   obstructive sleep *see* obstructive sleep apnoea
apnoea–hypopnea index (AHI) 95q, 104a
apoptosis 144q, 152a
arcuate eminence 31q, 42a

aspirin overdose 29q, 40a
audiological symbols 161q, 168a
audiometry
   play 166a
   pure tone 167a
   speech 27q, 39–40a
   visual reinforcement 33q, 43a, 166a, 192a
auditory brainstem implant
   indications 34q, 43a
   neurofibromatosis type 2 25q, 38a
auditory brainstem response (ABR) 26q, 39a, 163q, 169a
autosomal recessive inheritance 10q, 21a

B

bacteria 5q, 18a
barotrauma, flying-related 33q, 42a
basal cell carcinoma (BCC)
   clinical presentation 200q, 206–7a
   excision margins 117q, 129a
   forms 197q, 205a
   lower lip 116q
   multiple 143q, 151a
   nasal tip 116q, 129a
   risk factors 114q, 128a
basal skull fractures 14q, 23a
bat ear deformities 93q, 103a
Behçet syndrome 145q, 152a, 178q, 183a, 201q, 207a
Bell's palsy
   prognosis 32q, 42a
   synkinesis 157q, 164a
benign paroxysmal positional vertigo (BPPV)
   nystagmus 36q, 45a
   surgical treatment 38a
beta-2 transferrin 28q, 40a, 135a
bilobed (Zitelli) flap, dorsum of nose 117q, 129a
Bing–Sibenman malformation 41a
Bing's test 44a
bipolar electrosurgery 12q, 22a
blood supply
   carotid body tumour 51q, 75a
   reconstructive flaps 116q, 121q, 129a, 134a
   tonsils 14q, 23a, 66q, 82a
blood transfusion
   incorrect 4q, 17a
   refusal 90q, 101a
blood volume
   2-year-old child 94q, 103a
   loss, post-tonsillectomy haemorrhage 89q, 101a
bone-anchored hearing aids (BAHA) 33q, 42a
Borrelia burgdorferi 152a
botulinum toxin (Botox) 7q, 19a, 122q, 135a
   synkinesis 157q, 164a
Bowen disease 200q, 206–7a
brachycephaly 97q, 105a, 189q, 194a
branchial arches
   derivatives 186q, 192a
   first see first branchial arch

second see second branchial arch
   third and fourth 95q, 104a
branchial cleft fistula, first 87q, 100a
branchial cyst 74a
branchio-oto-renal (BOR) syndrome 44a, 95q, 104a, 126a
breathing, child with noisy 189q, 194a
bronchoscope, rigid 176q, 182a
bronchoscopy
   inhaled foreign body 103a, 189q, 194a
   vascular compression during 92q, 103a
   see also microlaryngoscopy and bronchoscopy (MLB),
     paediatric
Brown sign 161q, 168a
brown tumours 151a
Brun sign 161q
buccal nerve 16a
bulla ethmoidalis 203q, 209a
bupivacaine with adrenaline 147q, 154a

C

cancer
   clinical drug trials 7q, 19a
   performance status (PS) 83–84a
   treatment waiting times 9q, 20a
candida infection 64q, 81a
candidosis, chronic hyperplastic 180a
Canestan 162q, 168a
capillary vascular malformation, cutaneous 92q, 102a
carbimazole, side effects 9q, 21a, 63q, 80a
carbon dioxide (CO_2) laser 11q, 21a
Carhart's effect 33q, 42–43a
carotid body tumour, blood supply 51q, 75a
cavernous sinus
   anatomy 9q, 20a
   nasopharyngeal carcinoma extension 47q, 73a
   thrombosis 120q, 133–34a
cDNA microarrays 145q, 152a
cell biology 144q, 152a
cell cycle 11q, 22a
cellulitis, orbital 120q, 133–34a
cerebellopontine angle tumour 30q, 41a
cerebrospinal fluid (CSF) leaks 121q, 135a
   functional endoscopic sinus surgery 108q, 125a
   head injury 28q, 40a
   MRI features 110q, 126a
cervical lymphadenopathy, child with persistent 96q, 104a
cervical lymph node metastases see lymph node
   metastases
cervical vestibular evoked myogenic potentials
   (cVEMPs) 35q, 44a
Chagas disease 177q, 182a
CHARGE syndrome 102a, 104a
cheek
   basal cell carcinoma excision 117q, 129a
   swelling, CT scan 124q, 137a
chest X-rays see X-rays
Chevalier–Jackson sign 77a

children
blood volume calculation 94q, 103a
drug doses 185q, 187q, 192a
facial lacerations, closure 113a, 127a
fluid management 103a
sinonasal malignancies 199q, 206a
soft tissue malignancies 90q, 101a
subjective hearing tests 159q, 166–67a
upper respiratory tract infections 94q, 104a
see also neonates; paediatric otolaryngology
choanal atresia 91q, 102a, 122q, 135a
choking, child with history of 93–94q, 103a
cholesteatoma 33q, 43a, 159q, 167a
cholesterol granuloma 31q, 41a
chondrosarcoma 202q, 208a
chorda tympani
anatomy 16a, 157q, 164a
entry to infratemporal fossa 173q, 180–81a
chordomas
clival 32q, 42a
postnasal space 151a
chronic rhinosinusitis (CRS) 123q, 136a
Churg–Strauss syndrome see granulomatosis with polyangiitis
(GPA), with eosinophilia
Chvostek sign 7q, 19a
chylous fistula 48q, 73a
cilia, nasal 107q, 125a
ciliary dyskinesia, primary 126a
clinical trials
anticancer drugs 7q, 19a
design 14q, 23a
levels of evidence 10q, 21a
randomization 5q, 18a
clival chordomas 32q, 42a
Clostridium spp. 5q, 11q, 18a, 22a
clotting tests 149q, 156a
cocaine
abuse 203q, 209a
local anaesthesia 122q, 135a, 147q, 154a
cochlea
anatomy and physiology 26q, 39a
aplasia 41a
cochlear duct, partial aplasia 41a
cochlear hydrops 158q, 165a
cochlear implants 45a
Cogan syndrome 145q, 152a, 167a, 201q, 207a
collaural fistula 87q
complaints, handling 9q, 21a
computed tomography (CT)
cholesteatoma recurrence 33q, 43a
double density sign 107q, 125a
Lund–Mackay grading of sinus opacification 111q,
126–27a
pulsatile tinnitus 29q, 41a
congenital deafness
congenital cytomegalovirus 98q, 105a
with goitre 89q, 101a

histopathological findings 30q, 41a
imaging findings 96q
infectious aetiology 187q, 193a
investigations, sick neonates 96q, 104a
syndromes causing sensorineural 190q, 195a
congenital laryngeal webs 98q, 105a
congenital midline nasal lesions 119q, 132a
consent, parental responsibility 88q, 100a
Control of Noise at Work Regulations (2005) 40a
Converse technique 167a
cordectomy, transoral 68q, 83a
coronal suture, premature fusion 189q
cortical evoked response (CER) audiometry 26q, 39a
cough, persistent 70q, 85a
cranial sutures 186q, 192a
craniofacial abnormalities 189q, 194a
craniosynostosis 97q, 105a
cranial sutures 186q, 192a
frequency of different types 194a
CREST syndrome 23a, 182a
cribriform plate, clear fluid flowing from lateral
lamella 108q, 125a
Crohn disease 84a
croup, recurrent 99q, 105a
Crouzon syndrome
clinical features 188q, 193–94a
craniofacial abnormality 194a
craniosynostosis 97q, 105a
gene mutation 188q, 194a
CSF see cerebrospinal fluid
CT see computed tomography
cysts
branchial 74a
dermoid 105a, 132a
right anterior triangle of neck 49q, 74a
second branchial arch 59q, 78a
thyroglossal duct 59q, 79a
cytomegalovirus infection 98q, 105a
cytoplasmic antineutrophil cytoplasmic antibodies
(cANCA) 126a, 131–32a, 205a

D

dabigatran 22a
dark field microscopy 145q, 152–53a
deafness see hearing loss
decibel scale 40a
delayed endolymphatic hydrops 158q, 165a
delta sign, empty 150a
deltopectoral flap 134a, 174q, 181a
denture stomatitis 81a, 172q, 179a
dermoid cysts, nasal 105a, 132a
descendens hypoglossi nerve 16a, 174q, 181a
desmoglein antibodies 201q, 207a
developmental delay, hearing tests 185q, 192a
diplopia, nasal obstruction with 47q, 73a
diving 32q, 42a
DNA (deoxyribonucleic acid) 7q, 19–20a

double density sign 107q, 125a
Down syndrome
    associated features 92q, 102a
    hearing aid choice 162q, 168a
    prenatal markers 110q, 126a
driving, obstructive sleep apnoea 52q, 76a
drooling, child with persistent 98q, 105a
drop attacks 158q, 165a
drugs
    ear medications 162q, 168a
    idiosyncratic reactions 178q, 182–83a
    paediatric dosing 185q, 187q, 192a
dufourmentel flap 129a
dysphagia 70q, 85a
dysphonia, spasmodic 66q, 82a
dysplastic nevus syndrome 127a
dystopia canthorum 36q, 44a, 102a, 195a

E

Eagle syndrome 78a
ear
    development 88q, 100–1a
    medications 162q, 168a
ear protectors 27q, 40a
electrocardiogram (ECG), hypercalcaemia 6q, 19a
electrocochleography 26q, 39a
electromyography, laryngeal 68q, 83a
empty delta sign 150a
encephalocoeles 132a
endolymph
    electrolyte composition 26q, 39a
    flow after clockwise rotation 26q, 39a
endolymphatic hydrops, delayed 158q, 165a
endoscopic assessment of swallow, modified
        flexible 70q, 85a
endoscopic transethmoidal sphenoidotomy 107q, 125a
endotracheal intubation, newborn infant 99q, 105–6a
endotracheal tubes, paediatric 187q, 193a
energy calculations, children 187q, 193a
epiglottis, thumb-printing 150a
epiglottitis 189q, 194a
epistaxis
    catheters for postnasal packing 109q, 126a
    causes 198q, 206a
    clotting tests 149q, 156a
epithelia 178q, 182a
Epstein–Barr virus (EBV)-negative tumour, unknown
        primary 72q, 86a
erythroplakia 178q, 182a
esthesioneuroblastoma see olfactory neuroblastoma
ethmoidal air cells, endoscopic removal 108q, 125a
ethmoidectomy, external 108q, 125a
ethmoid sinus adenocarcinoma see sinonasal adenocarcinoma
Eustachian tube, muscles opening 87q, 100a
evidence, levels 10q, 21a, 147q, 153a
Ewald's first law 36q, 44a
Ewald's second and third laws 44a

exostoses 157q, 164a
external auditory canal
    atresia, isolated 88q, 100–1a
    cartilagenous portion 34q, 43a
    osteoma 31q, 42a
    paraesthesia 30q, 41a
    sinus opening into 87q, 100a
external carotid artery, branches 177q, 182a
external ear see outer ear
external nasal nerve 136a

F

face
    aesthetic analysis 113q, 121q, 127a, 134a, 200q, 207a
    ageing 122q, 135a
    lacerations, closure in children 113q, 127a
    reanimation techniques 68q, 83a, 157q, 164a
    wound healing 114q, 128a
facial nerve
    branches 16a
    identification during parotidectomy 47q, 73a
    internal auditory meatus relations 35q, 44a
    preservation, parotid tumours 86a
    sural nerve interposition cable graft 115q, 128a
facial nerve palsy
    after modified radical mastoidectomy 28q, 40a
    child with parotid mass 90q, 101a
    diagnosis of cause 144q, 151–52a
    facial reanimation techniques 68q, 83a, 157q, 164a
    House–Brackmann grade IV 32q, 42a
factor assays 149q, 156a
familial adenomatous polyposis 132a
fascia lata sling 164a
fibroblast growth factor receptor (FGFR)-related
        craniosynostosis 105a
fibroblasts, wound healing 115q, 128a
fibrous dysplasia 143q, 151a
fibula free flap 134a
fine needle aspiration (FNA) of neck mass
    normal thyroid cells 57q, 78a
    unknown primary 80a
fine needle aspiration (FNA) of thyroid
    follicular thyroid carcinoma 49q, 74a
    possible follicular neoplasm 56q, 77a
    Thy 2 thyroid nodule 49q, 74a
    Thy 3 thyroid nodule 53q
first branchial arch 94q, 104a
    derivatives 4q, 17a
fissures of Santorini 157q, 164a
Fitzpatrick skin types 128a
flaps 117q, 129a
    Abbe 116q, 128–29a
    arterial supply 116q, 121q, 129a, 134a
    bilobed (Zitelli) 117q, 129a
    delayed division of pedicle 116q, 128–29a
    rhomboid rotational 115q, 128a
    selection 174q, 181a

flexible endoscopic assessment of swallowing (FEES) 70q, 85a
fluid challenge, children 103a, 185q, 192a
fluid maintenance, children 103a
fluoroquinolones 151a
flying, barotrauma following 33q, 42a
follicular thyroid carcinoma
    diagnosis 49q, 74a
    incidence 49q, 74a
    postoperative complications 54q, 77a
follicular thyroid neoplasm, possible 56q, 77a
food bolus obstruction 51q, 75a
foramen ovale 173q, 180a
foramina 173q, 180–81a
Fordyce spots 80a
foreign bodies
    ingested 60q, 79a
    inhaled 93–94q, 103a, 189q, 194a
    nasal cavity 198q, 206a
Foster Kennedy syndrome 202q, 208a
Frankfurt plane 134a
French catheter scale 109q, 126a
Frey syndrome 83a
frontal recess 112q, 127a
frontal sinus, development 110q, 123q, 126a, 136a
functional endoscopic sinus surgery (FESS) 108q, 125a
fungal sinusitis 123q, 136a
    allergic 125a
Furstenberg test 97q, 105a, 132a
Fusobacterium necrophorum 75a

G
Gardasil vaccine 89q, 101a
Gell and Coombs classification 8q, 20a, 201q, 207a
gene microarrays 145q, 152a
general otolaryngology 3q, 16q, 141q, 150q
genetics
    autosomal recessive conditions 10q, 21a
    neurofibromatosis type 2 28q, 40a, 43a
    paediatric syndromes 188q, 194a
    vagal paraganglioma 37q, 45a
    see also inheritance
gentamicin, ototoxicity 32q, 42a
geographical tongue 81a
Gillies fan flap 129a
gingival hyperplasia 172q, 179a
glabella 200q, 207a
Glaserian fissure (petrotympanic fissure) 173q, 180–81a
gliomas, nasal 132a
glomus tympanicum tumour 168a
glossopharyngeal nerve 16a
goitre
    investigations 53q, 76a
    Pendred syndrome 89q, 101a, 190q, 195a
Gorlin syndrome 92q, 103a, 151a
Gradenigo syndrome 35q, 43a
granulomatosis with polyangiitis (GPA) 110q, 126a, 131–32a
    with eosinophilia 131–32a, 205a

nasal crusting 198q, 205a
nasal septal perforation 203q, 209a
posterior pharyngeal wall lesion 151a
granulomatous disorders
    Gell and Coombs classification 201q, 207a
    nose 119q, 131–32a
Graves disease
    orbital decompression 56q, 78a
    thyroidectomy counselling 59q, 79a
greater superficial petrosal nerve 16a, 174q, 181a
Griesinger sign 161q
Guillain–Barré syndrome (GBS) 144q, 152a
gunshot wound, facial nerve palsy 157q, 164a
gustatory sweating, post parotidectomy 67q, 83a

H
haemangiomas
    cutaneous 91q, 102a
    subglottic 97q, 102a, 105a
haematomas
    sternocleidomastoid muscle 88q, 100a
    vocal cord 48q, 73a
haemorrhage, post-tonsillectomy 89q, 90q, 101a
haemostasis, surgical 12q, 22a
hand, foot and mouth disease 186q, 193a
Hansen disease (leprosy) 201q, 207a
hardwood exposure 127a, 199q, 206a
Hashimoto disease (chronic lymphocytic thyroiditis) 171q, 179a
head and neck surgery 47q, 73a, 171q, 179a
head injury 28q, 40a
hearing aids
    bone-anchored (BAHA) 33q, 42a
    selection 162q, 168a
hearing loss
    aspirin overdose 29q, 40a
    branchio-oto-renal syndrome 95q, 104a
    Carhart's effect 42–43a
    cerebellopontine angle tumour 30q, 41a
    congenital see congenital deafness
    cytomegalovirus infection 98q, 105a
    dystopia canthorum with sensorineural 36q, 44a
    gentamicin toxicity 42a
    imaging in paediatric 96q, 104a
    investigation of paediatric 185q, 192a
    noise-induced 27q, 40a
    non-organic, tests for 35q, 44a
    osteoma-related 31q, 42a
    paediatric infections 187q, 193a
    SCUBA diver 32q, 42a
    syndromic 160q, 167a
    vertigo with 158q, 165a
    windsurfer with fluctuating 36q, 45a
hearing protectors 27q, 40a
hearing tests
    sick neonates 96q, 104a
    subjective, for children 159q, 166–67a
    see also audiometry

Heerfordt syndrome 201q, 207a
Hennebert sign 161q, 168a
hereditary haemorrhagic telangiectasia
    (Osler–Weber–Rendu syndrome) 120q, 134a
    epistaxis 198q, 206a
hiatus semilunaris 203q, 209a
Hirschsprung disease 190q, 195a
histological diagnoses 143q, 151a
Hitselberger sign 41a, 161q, 168a
HIV infection 8q, 20a
hoarseness
    infant intubated at birth 99q, 105–6a
    microlaryngoscopy 65q, 82a
    occasional, with laryngeal oedema 53q, 76a
Holman–Miller sign 132–33a
homocystinuria 93q, 103a
human papillomaviruses (HPV)
    mechanism of carcinogenesis 69q, 84a
    negative tumours, TNM staging 72q, 86a
    positive tonsillar carcinoma, staging 69q, 84a
    recurrent respiratory papillomatosis
        subtypes 89q, 101a
    vaccination 89q, 101a
hyoid bone 5q, 18a
hypercalcaemia
    ECG abnormalities 6q, 19a
    parathyroid tumour localization 58q, 78a
hyperfractionated radiotherapy 63q, 80a
hyperparathyroidism
    localization of overactive parathyroid 65q, 82a
    medullary thyroid carcinoma and RET
        mutations 52q, 75a
    primary 143q, 151a
hyperplasia 146q, 153a
hypersensitivity reactions 201q, 207a
hypertension, obstructive sleep apnoea 52q, 76a
hypertrophy 146q, 153a
hypocalcaemia
    clinical features 77a
    permanent post thyroidectomy 65q, 82a
hypoglossal facial anastomosis 164a
hypoglossal nerve, identification 47q, 73a
hypomagnesaemia 19a
hypopharyngeal tumours 55q, 77a
    T staging 59q, 79a
hypopharynx 55q, 77a
hypotension, intraoperative 60q, 79a
hypothyroidism 61q, 79a

I
ibuprofen, paediatric dose 185q, 192a
imaging
    choice of modality 159q, 167a
    cholesteatoma recurrence 33q
    cholesterol granuloma 31q, 41a
    paediatric hearing loss 96q, 104a
    parapharyngeal lesion 62q, 80a
    parathyroid tumour localization 58q, 78a
    radiological signs 141q, 150a
    see also computed tomography; magnetic resonance
        imaging; ultrasound; X-rays
immunoglobulins 5q, 18a
immunohistochemistry, P16 71q, 86a
incus, development 4q, 17a
induction of anaesthesia, child with history of
        choking 94q, 103a
infections
    aetiology 142q, 150a
    childhood hearing loss 187q, 193a
    paediatric 186q, 193a
    paediatric upper respiratory tract 94q, 104a
infectious diseases, systemic 201q, 207a
inferior alveolar nerve 23a
inferior vestibular nerve 38a
inflammatory bowel disease 84a
inflammatory diseases, systemic 201q, 207a
inheritance
    autosomal recessive 10q, 21a
    neurofibromatosis type 2 28q, 40a
    paediatric syndromes 190q, 195a
    see also genetics
injection thyroplasty 67q, 83a
inner ear
    development 160q, 168a
    diving-related injury 32q, 42a
    gentamicin toxicity 32q, 42a
inner hair cells 26q, 39a
internal auditory meatus 35q, 44a
internal carotid artery, branches 15q, 24a
internal jugular vein
    inadvertent puncture 64q, 81a
    spinal accessory nerve relations 52q, 75a
    thrombosis 50q, 75a
inverted papilloma 120q, 133a
    malignant transformation 130–31a
    unilateral nasal obstruction 112q, 127a
iron deficiency anaemia 77a

J
Jacobsen's nerve 83a
Jehovah's Witnesses 90q, 101a
Jervell–Lange-Nielsen syndrome 190q, 195a
jugular foramen
    lesions, nerve involvement 29q, 40a
    spinal accessory nerve 173q, 180a
juvenile nasal angiofibroma 49q, 74a, 120q, 132–33a
    clinical presentation 199q, 206a
    management 109q, 125–26a

K
Kallmann syndrome 135a, 202q, 208a
Karapandzic flap 129a
Kartagener syndrome 126a
Kawasaki disease 186q, 193a

Klebsiella rhinoscleromatis 198*q*, 205*a*
knife wounds
    face 114*q*, 128*a*
    neck 50*q*, 74–75*a*
Koerner's septum 25*q*, 38*a*
Kruskal–Wallis test 156*a*

L

labrale inferius 200*q*, 207*a*
labyrinth
    dysplasia of membranous 41*a*
    incomplete development 41*a*
    ossification of bony 34*q*, 43*a*
labyrinthine artery 38*a*
lacquers, exposure to 202*q*, 208*a*
Lancefield group C streptococci 5*q*, 18*a*
laryngeal carcinoma
    postoperative radiotherapy 60*q*, 79*a*
    spread to pre-epiglottic space 55*q*, 77*a*
    T1a mid-cord, initial management 71*q*, 86*a*
    T2, transoral resection 68*q*, 83*a*
laryngeal muscles, intrinsic 10*q*, 21*a*
laryngeal oedema
    drainage 54*q*, 76*a*
    smoker with voice changes 53*q*, 76*a*
laryngeal webs, congenital 98*q*, 105*a*
laryngectomy
    hypoglossal nerve identification 47*q*, 73*a*
    postoperative radiotherapy 60*q*, 79*a*
laryngocele, internal 85*a*
laryngomalacia 87*q*, 91*q*, 100*a*, 102*a*
larynx
    development 91*q*, 102*a*
    electromyography 68*q*, 83*a*
lasers 5*q*, 17*a*, 175*q*, 181*a*
    carbon dioxide (CO_2) 11*q*, 21*a*
Lemierre syndrome 75*a*
leprosy 201*q*, 207*a*
Lermoyez syndrome 44*a*, 158*q*, 165*a*
lesser petrosal nerve 16*a*, 173*q*, 174*q*, 180*a*, 181*a*
lethal midline granuloma 203*q*, 209*a*
leucoplakia 179*a*, 182*a*
    chronic hyperplastic 81*a*
leucoplasia, proliferative verrucous 172*q*, 179*a*
Lhermitte sign 83*a*
lidocaine
    with adrenaline, safe dose 13*q*, 23*a*, 147*q*, 154*a*
    mechanism of action 135*a*
    without adrenaline, safe dose 108*q*, 125*a*
Lignospan, safe dose 13*q*, 23*a*
lingual erythema migrans 81*a*
lingual nerve 16*a*
local anaesthesia 123*q*, 136*a*
local anaesthetics 122*q*, 135*a*
    pharmacokinetics 4*q*, 17*a*
    safe doses 13*q*, 23*a*, 108*q*, 125*a*
    volume and dose calculations 147*q*, 154*a*

lorazepam, paediatric dose 187*q*, 193*a*
lower lateral cartilages 204*q*, 209*a*
lower lip tumours 115*q*, 128*a*
    basal cell carcinoma 116*q*, 129*a*
    squamous cell carcinoma 175*q*, 181*a*
Lund–Mackay scoring system 111*q*, 126–27*a*, 136*a*
lupus pernio 131–32*a*, 200*q*, 206–7*a*
Lyme disease 144*q*, 152*a*
lymph node biopsy
    local anaesthesia 108*q*, 125*a*
    sentinel 84–85*a*, 86*a*
lymph node metastases
    lower lip tumours 128*a*
    nasopharyngeal carcinoma, staging 57*q*, 78*a*
    tonsillar carcinoma 48*q*, 73*a*
    with unknown primary, TNM staging 72*q*, 86*a*
lymph nodes
    nasal cavity first-echelon 48*q*, 73*a*
    thyroid tissue in 78*a*

M

magnetic resonance imaging (MRI)
    acoustic neuroma 159*q*, 167*a*
    cerebellopontine angle tumour 30*q*, 41*a*
    cholesterol granuloma 31*q*, 41*a*
    CSF rhinorrhoea 110*q*, 126*a*
    nasal mass 109*q*, 125–26*a*
    recurrent cholesteatoma 33*q*, 43*a*, 159*q*, 167*a*
malleus, development 4*q*, 17*a*
mandibular nerve, sensory branches 13*q*, 23*a*
mandibulotomy, paramedian 64*q*, 81*a*
mastoid process, muscle attachments 4*q*, 17*a*
maxillary sinus
    antrochoanal polyps 133*a*
    development 110*q*, 126*a*
    double density sign 107*q*, 125*a*
maxillary sinus (squamous cell) carcinoma
    first-echelon nodes 48*q*, 73*a*
    Ohngren's line 108*q*, 125*a*
    T staging 109*q*, 126*a*, 199*q*, 206*a*
McCune–Albright syndrome 151*a*
measles 187*q*, 193*a*
Meckel's cartilage 104*a*
median rhomboid glossitis 81*a*
medullary thyroid carcinoma (MTC)
    hyperparathyroidism and *RET*
        mutations 52*q*, 75*a*
    management 58*q*, 78*a*
    origin 49*q*, 74*a*
    prognosis of MEN 2B-associated 49*q*, 74*a*
    prophylactic surgery 81*a*, 105*a*
melanoma, malignant 113*q*, 127–28*a*
    AJCC staging 114*q*, 128*a*
    cutaneous 119*q*, 131*a*
    mucosal sinonasal 118*q*, 130–31*a*, 199*q*, 206*a*
    recurrent 69*q*, 84–85*a*
Melkersson–Rosenthal syndrome 144*q*, 151–52*a*

Ménière disease 35q, 44a
  electrocochleography 26q, 39a
  probable 158q, 165a
menton 200q, 207a
merlin protein 43a
metaplasia 146q, 153a
Michel aplasia 36q, 41a, 45a
microlaryngoscopy
  persistent cough 70q, 85a
  smoker with hoarseness 65q, 82a
microlaryngoscopy and bronchoscopy (MLB), paediatric
  anaesthesia 95q, 104a
  infant intubated at birth 99q, 105–6a
  subglottic haemangioma 97q, 105a
microtia 90q, 101a
middle cranial fossa
  approach, acoustic neuroma 25q, 38a
  arcuate eminence 31q, 42a
middle ear
  sound-transformer mechanisms 31q, 42a
  testing, tympanometry 159q, 166a
midline nasal lesions, congenital 119q, 132a
Moh's micrographic surgery 117q, 129a
molecular biology techniques 145q, 152a
Mondini malformation 41a, 43a
monopolar electrosurgery 12q, 22a
morphine sulphate, paediatric dose 185q, 192a
motor nerves 141q, 150a
MRI see magnetic resonance imaging
mucoceles 123q, 136a
mucoepidermoid carcinoma, parotid 173q, 180a
  low grade 72q, 86a
  paediatric 101a
multidisciplinary team, voice clinic 54q, 77a
multiple endocrine neoplasia (MEN)
  paediatric management 98q, 105a
  prophylactic surgery 81–82a, 105a
  type 2A 75a
  type 2B 49q, 74a, 75a
multiple sleep latency test 76a
mumps, hearing loss 187q, 193a
muscles
  innervation anatomy 141q, 150a
  mastoid process attachments 4q, 17a
Mustardé technique 167a
mycobacteria, non-tuberculous (NTB) 96q, 104a,
  186q, 193a
Myer–Cotton grading, subglottic stenosis 91q, 102a

N

narrow-band imaging (NBI) 72q, 86a
nasal bone, traumatic injury 10q, 21a
nasal crusting 198q, 205a
nasal masses
  clinical scenarios 199q, 206a
  infant with enlarging 97q, 105a
  MRI scan 109q, 125–26a
  see also nasal tumours

nasal obstruction
  CT scanning 107q, 124q, 125a, 137a
  diplopia with 47q, 73a
  investigations for unilateral 112q, 127a
  supraclavicular mass with 57q, 78a
nasal septal perforation see septal perforation
nasal tip
  projection 127q, 134a
  repair, after tumour excision 116q, 129a
  sensory innervation 10q, 21a
  support mechanisms 121q, 134a
nasal tumours 202q, 208a
  inverted papilloma 120q, 133a
  juvenile angiofibroma see juvenile nasal
    angiofibroma
  see also nasal masses; sinonasal malignancies
nasal wall (lateral), osteology 108q
nasendoscopy, flexible 189q, 194a
nasolabial angle 127a
nasopharyngeal carcinoma 118q, 130a
  cavernous sinus extension 47q, 73a
  initial management 51q, 75a
  staging of neck disease 57q, 78a
  T staging 199q, 206a
neck dissection
  chylous fistula after 48q, 73a
  internal jugular vein ligation 52q, 75a
  internal jugular vein puncture 64q, 81a
  intraoperative complications 60q, 79a
  parotid tumours 86a
  postoperative radiotherapy 60q, 79a
  T1 oral carcinoma 71q, 85–86a
neck injuries, penetrating 50q, 74–75a
neck masses
  cyst in right anterior triangle 49q, 74a
  fine needle aspiration (FNA) 57q, 78a, 80a
  histological diagnoses 143q, 151a
  investigations 63q, 80a
  newborn baby 88q, 100a
  with solitary enlarged lymph node 48q, 73a
  thyroglossal duct cyst 59q, 79a
neck pain, child with homocystinuria 93q, 103a
needles, surgical 123q, 136a
negative predictive value 18a
neonates
  intubated at birth 99q, 105–6a
  investigation of hearing loss 185q
  neck mass 88q, 100a
nerve injury
  left nasal bone trauma 10q, 21a
  modified radical mastoidectomy 28q, 40a
  superior laryngeal nerve 59q, 79a
nerves
  head and neck 174q, 181a
  jugular foramen 29q, 40a
  motor 141q, 150a
  superior orbital fissure 4q, 17a
nerve sheath tumours, parapharyngeal space 80a

neurofibromatosis type 2 (NF2)
  auditory brainstem implant 25q, 38–39a
  genetics 28q, 40a
  protein associated with 34q, 43a
neuro-otology 25q, 38a, 157q, 164a
newborn hearing screening programme (NHSP) 96q, 104a, 192a
new oral anticoagulants 11q, 22a
Nikolsky sign 201q, 207a
noise exposure, occupational 27q, 40a
noise-induced hearing loss 27q, 40a
non-Hodgkin lymphoma, T-cell type 203q, 209a
non-tuberculous mycobacteria (NTB) 96q, 104a, 186q, 193a
nose
  aesthetic units 114q, 128a
  ciliary physiology and anatomy 107q, 125a
  congenital midline lesions 119q, 132a
  dorsum, bilobed (Zitelli) flap 117q, 129a
  embryology 110q, 126a, 132a
  granulomatous disorders 119q, 131–32a
  lateral nasal wall osteology 108q, 125a
  tumours see nasal tumours
nystagmus
  benign paroxysmal positional vertigo 36q, 45a
  diagnosis of type 158q, 166a
  Ewald's first law 36q, 44a
  right fast beating 26q, 39a

O

obesity
  local anaesthetic dose 13q, 23a
obstructive sleep apnoea (OSA) 52q, 76a, 118q, 130a
  male HGV driver 52q, 76a
  paediatric 95q, 98q, 104a, 105a, 191q, 195a
odontogenic lesions 143q, 151a
odynophagia 85a, 189q, 194a
oesophageal carcinoma 177q, 182a
oesophageal disorders 14q, 23a, 177q, 182a
oesophageal obstruction 51q, 75a
oesophagoscopy, rigid 51q, 75a
Ohngren's line 108q, 125a
olfaction
  ammonia 110q, 126a, 135a
  disorders 121q, 135a
  physiology 3q, 17a
  see also anosmia
olfactory neuroblastoma 130–31a, 202q, 208a
opera singer 48q, 73a
optic canal 7q, 20a
oral candida infection 64q, 81a
oral cavity carcinoma
  diagnosis 172q, 179–80a
  T1, management 71q, 85–86a
  TNM staging 71q, 86a
  see also tongue carcinoma; tonsillar carcinoma
oral disease
  associations 69q, 84a
  diagnosis 172q, 179–80a
oral stomatitis 81a

oral ulceration
  pemphigus vulgaris 201q, 207a
  persistent 63q, 80a
  traumatic 172q, 179a
orbital apex syndrome 123q, 136a
orbital cavity, bones 110q, 126a
orbital cellulitis 120q, 133–34a
orbital decompression, thyroid eye disease 56q, 78a
Osler–Weber–Rendu disease see hereditary haemorrhagic
      telangiectasia
ossicular chain development 4q, 17a, 168a
osteoma
    common sites 157q, 164a
    ear canal 31q, 42a
otalgia, referred 3q, 16a
otitis externa, recurrent 36q, 45a
otitis media, contraindicating
      stapedotomy 40a
otoacoustic emissions (OAEs) 27q, 39a, 167a
otology 25q, 38a, 157q, 164a
Otomize 162q, 168a
otosclerosis 34q, 43a
    infectious aetiology 187q, 193a
    sodium fluoride therapy 31q, 41a
Otosporin 162q, 168a
otosyphilis 161q, 168a
outer ear
    bat ear deformities 93q, 103a
    pinnal growth 34q, 43a
    sound-transformer mechanisms 31q, 42a
outer hair cells
    anatomy 26q, 39a
    noise-induced damage 40a
    otoacoustic emissions 39a

P

P16-positive tumours 71q, 86a
p53 protein 84a
paediatric otolaryngology 87q, 100a, 185q, 192a
    see also children; neonates
papillary thyroid carcinoma
    incidence 49q, 74a
    metastatic well-differentiated 78a
    thyroglossal duct cyst 59q, 79a
papillomatosis, respiratory see respiratory papillomatosis
paracetamol, paediatric dose 185q, 192a
paracusis Willisii 161q
paraesthesia, ear canal 30q, 41a
paragangliomas 151a
    vagal 37q, 45a
paramedian mandibulotomy 64q, 81a
paranasal sinuses
    CT scanning 107q, 125a
    development 103a
    embryology 110q, 126a
    functional endoscopic sinus surgery 108q, 125a
    fungal disease 123q, 136a
    Lund–Mackay grading 111q, 126–27a, 136a

paranasal sinus tumours 202q, 208a
  see also maxillary sinus carcinoma; sinonasal malignancies
parapharyngeal space
  anatomy 55q, 77a
  lesions 61q, 62q, 80a
parasympathetic nerves
  saliva production 16a
  submandibular gland 3q, 16a
parathyroid gland, localization of overactive 65q, 82a
parathyroid hormone 8q, 20a
  intraoperative monitoring 82a
  post thyroidectomy 82a
parathyroid tumours, imaging 58q, 78a
parental responsibility 88q, 100a
parotidectomy
  facial nerve identification 47q, 73a
  gustatory sweating after 67q, 83a
parotid fistula 49q, 74a
parotid gland, saliva production 16a
parotid tumours
  malignant paediatric 90q, 101a
  mucoepidermoid carcinoma 72q, 86a, 101a, 173q, 180a
  pleomorphic adenoma 49q, 74a
  pregnancy 64q, 81a
  salivary duct carcinoma 173q, 180a
pars tensa, development 34q, 43a
patent ductus arteriosus (PDA), surgery for 99q, 105–6a
Patterson–Kelly–Brown syndrome 77a
pectoralis major flap, Poland syndrome 174q, 181a
pemphigoid 183a, 207a
pemphigus 84a, 178q, 183a, 201q, 207a
Pendred syndrome 89q, 101a
  diagnostic features 158q, 165a, 167a, 190q, 195a
  hearing loss type 44a
  Mondini malformation 41a
  pendrin protein 12q, 22a
penicillins 22a, 151a
perchlorate test 101a
performance status (PS) 68q, 83–84a
perinuclear antineutrophil cytoplasmic antibodies
    (pANCA) 126a, 131–32a, 205a
petrotympanic fissure (Glaserian fissure) 173q, 180–81a
phase 1 trials 19a
phase 2 trials 19a
phase 3 trials 19a
Phelp sign 157q, 164a
pinna, growth 34q, 43a
pinnaplasty 160q, 167a
plasmacytoma 85a
platelet count 8q, 20a, 149q, 156a
play audiometry 166a
pleomorphic adenoma 49q, 74a
Plummer–Vinson syndrome 77a
Poiseuille's law 101a
Poisson regression 156a
Poland syndrome 174q, 181a
polymerase chain reaction (PCR) 145q, 152a

polypropylene sutures 146q, 153a
port wine stain 102a
positive predictive value 18a
positron emission tomography–computed tomography (PET-
    CT) scan, neck masses 80a
positron emission tomography (PET)-FDG scanning 51q, 75a
post-cricoid squamous cell carcinoma 55q, 77a
posterior cricoarytenoid muscle 21a
posterior ethmoidal artery 108q, 125a
posterior pharyngeal wall lesion 143q, 151a
postnasal space
  biopsy 143q, 151a
  mass 51q, 75a
postpartum thyroiditis 171q, 179a
preauricular sinuses 95q, 104a
pre-epiglottic space, laryngeal carcinoma spread 55q, 77a
pregnancy, parotid acinic cell carcinoma 64q, 81a
prevalence 18a
pre-vertebral soft tissues, widening 150a
prion diseases 8q, 20a
prophylactic surgery, RET mutation carriers 64q,
    81–82a, 105a
propranolol, for subglottic haemangioma 97q, 105a
pterygopalatine fossa
  nasal lesion involving 109q, 125–26a
  tumours 50q, 75a
pulsed dye laser 181a
pulse oximetry, obstructive sleep apnoea 76a
pure tone audiometry 167a
p-value 6q, 19a
pyogenic granuloma 198q, 199q, 206a
pyostomatitis vegetans 84a
pyriform fossa tumour, T staging 59q, 79a
pyriform sinus, pooling of saliva 55q, 77a

Q
QT interval, prolonged 190q, 195a
quinolones 22a, 151a

R
radial forearm flap 129a
radical mastoidectomy, facial nerve palsy after 28q, 40a
radiographs see X-rays
radiological imaging see imaging
radiotherapy
  acute side effects 67q, 83a
  hyperfractionated 63q, 80a
  laryngeal carcinoma 60q, 79a
  tumour sensitivity 63q, 80a
radix 200q, 207a
randomization 5q, 18a
randomized controlled trials 10q, 21a
Rb protein 84a
reconstructive flaps see flaps
referred otalgia 3q, 16a
Reinke oedema 56q, 76a, 77a
relapsing perichondritis 201q, 207a

respiratory papillomatosis
  recurrent, HPV subtypes 89q, 101a
  smoker with hoarseness 82a
retinal flecks 190q, 195a
RET mutation carriers
  management of paediatric 98q, 105a
  medullary thyroid carcinoma and
    hyperparathyroidism 52q, 75a
  prophylactic surgery 64q, 81–82a, 105a
rhabdomyosarcoma
  nasal 199q, 202q, 206a, 208a
  relative frequency 101a
rheumatoid arthritis
  hearing aid choice 162q, 168a
  oral ulceration 63q, 80a
rhinion 200q, 207a
rhinology 107q, 125a, 197q, 205a
rhinoplasty
  anatomy 204q, 209a
  techniques 113q, 127a
rhinorrhoea
  bloody, CT scan 124q, 137a
  CSF see cerebrospinal fluid (CSF) leaks
  intermittent green 94q, 104a
  persistent purulent 95q, 104a
rhinoscleroma 198q, 205a
rhinosinusitis, chronic (CRS) 123q, 136a
rhinosporidiosis 198q, 205a
rhomboid rotational flap 115q, 128a
right subclavian artery, compression 92q, 103a
rivaroxaban 11q, 22a
RNA interference (RNAi) 20a, 144q, 152a
rotation, clockwise 26q, 39a
rubella, congenital 186q, 193a

S
saccule 38a
saliva 3q, 16a
salivary duct carcinoma 173q, 180a
salivary gland tumours 173q, 180a
  clinical features 175q, 181a
  nose and paranasal space 202q, 208a
  see also parotid tumours
sarcoidosis
  extrapulmonary manifestations 13q, 23a
  nasal crusting 198q, 205a
  septal perforation 203q, 209a
  upper airway 119q, 131–32a
scaphocephaly 189q, 194a
scars
  strength of facial 114q, 128a
  Z-plasty 114q, 128a
Scheibe malformation 41a
schizophrenia 202q, 208a
schwannoma 151a
Schwartze sign 161q
scleroderma 177q, 182a

screening tests 6q, 18a
SCUBA diver 32q, 42a
second branchial arch
  abnormalities, branchio-oto-renal syndrome 95q, 104a
  cyst 59q, 78a
sensitivity, test 18a
sentinel lymph node biopsy 84–85a, 86a
septal cartilage 204q, 209a
septal perforation
  anterior, management 113q, 127a
  causes 203q, 209a
  iatrogenic 198q, 205a
septic emboli 50q, 75a
shock
  intraoperative 60q, 79a
  paediatric, fluid management 103a
  type I 101a
sickle cell crisis 11q, 22a
signs
  clinical 161q, 168a
  radiological 141q, 150a
silk sutures 23a, 146q, 153a
silver nitrate cautery 12q, 22a
singers, professional
  possible follicular neoplasm 56q, 77a
  Thy 3 thyroid nodule 53q, 76a
  vocal cord haematoma 48q, 73a
sinonasal adenocarcinoma
  clinical presentation 199q, 206a
  risk factors 112q, 127a, 202q, 208a
  T staging 199q, 206a
sinonasal malignancies 118q, 130–31a, 202q, 208a
  clinical scenarios 199q, 206a
  T staging 199q, 206a
sinonasal tumours 202q, 208a
  see also nasal tumours; paranasal sinus tumours
sinuses
  below pinna 87q, 100a
  paranasal see paranasal sinuses
  preauricular 95q, 104a
sinusitis
  2-year-old child 94q, 103a
  allergic fungal 125a
  fungal 123q, 136a
Sjögren syndrome, primary 50q, 74a
skin cancer
  clinical presentation 200q, 206–7a
  non-melanomatous 119q, 131a
  see also basal cell carcinoma; melanoma; squamous cell
    carcinoma, cutaneous
skin disorders 178q, 182–83a
  clinical presentation 200q, 206–7a
skin grafts, full-thickness 116q, 117q, 128a, 129a
skin types, Fitzpatrick 128a
skull base
  anatomy 119q, 131a
  fractures 14q, 23a

smell, sense of see olfaction
smokers
    microlaryngoscopy for hoarseness 65q, 82a
    voice changes and laryngeal oedema 53q, 76a
sodium fluoride 31q, 41a
Sofradex 162q, 168a
soft tissue malignancies, childhood 90q, 101a
solar keratosis see actinic keratosis
sound-transformer mechanisms, outer and middle ear 31q, 42a
spasmodic dysphonia 66q, 82a
specificity, test 18a
speech audiometry 27q, 39–40a
speech delay, testing hearing 185q, 192a
sphenoidotomy, transethmoidal 107q, 125a
spinal accessory nerve
    internal jugular vein relations 52q, 75a
    jugular foramen 173q, 180a
squamous cell carcinoma (SCC)
    cutaneous 119q, 131a, 200q, 206–7a
    laryngeal see laryngeal carcinoma
    lower lip 175q, 181a
    maxillary sinus see maxillary sinus carcinoma
    post-cricoid region 55q, 77a
    postnasal space 51q, 75a
    sinonasal 199q, 206a
    tongue see tongue carcinoma
    tonsil see tonsillar carcinoma
standard deviation 156a
standard error 156a
stapedial artery, persistent 41a
stapedotomy, contraindications 28q, 40a
stapes, development 4q, 17a
statistical terms 148q, 156a
statistical testing 6q, 19a, 148q, 155a, 156a
steeple sign 141q, 150a
Stenström technique 167a
stereocilia 26q, 39a
sternocleidomastoid flap 129a, 174q, 181a
sternocleidomastoid muscle haematoma 88q, 100a
Stevens–Johnson syndrome 178q, 182–83a
streptococci, Lancefield group C 5q, 18a
Streptococcus milleri 150a
stria vascularis, hypoplasia 41a
stridor
    chronic 189q, 194a
    infant intubated at birth 99q, 105–6a
    inspiratory, 6-month-old child 97q
study design 14q, 23a
study types 146q, 153a
Sturge–Weber syndrome 102a
styloid process, elongated 78a
stylomandibular ligament 77a
subclavian artery, right, compression 92q, 103a
subglottic haemangiomas
    associated cutaneous lesions 102a
    management 97q, 105a

subglottic stenosis, Myer–Cotton
    grading 91q, 102a
submandibular gland
    cribriform adenoid cystic carcinoma 173q, 180a
    parasympathetic innervation 3q, 16a
subnasale 200q, 207a
substance abuse 203q, 209a
super-antigen theory 136a
superior laryngeal nerve 73a
    injury 59q, 79a
superior orbital fissure 4q, 17a
superior vestibular nerve 38a
supraclavicular flap 134a
supratip 200q, 207a
supratrochlear nerve 136a
sural nerve interposition graft 115q, 128a, 164a
suture materials 13q, 23a, 122q, 136a, 146q, 153a
swallowing
    endoscopic assessment 70q, 85a
    foreign body sensation on 60q, 79a
    mechanism 13q, 23a
synkinesis 157q, 164a
syphilis 131–32a, 145q, 152–53a, 161q, 168a
systemic lupus erythematosus (SLE) 172q, 179a

T
tachycardia, intraoperative 60q, 79a
target lesions, skin 178q, 183a
T-cell type non-Hodgkin lymphoma 203q, 209a
telangiectasia, hereditary haemorrhagic see hereditary
        haemorrhagic telangiectasia
temporal bone
    arcuate eminence 31q, 42a
    cholesterol granuloma 31q, 41a
    fracture, imaging 159q, 167a
    openings 25q, 38a
tensor veli palatini muscle 100a
textile workers 199q, 206a
throat discomfort, chronic right-sided 58q, 78a
thrombocytopenia 8q, 20a
thrombosis
    cavernous sinus 120q, 133–34a
    homocystinuria 103a
    internal jugular vein 50q, 75a
thyroglobulin, serum 76a
thyroglossal duct cyst 59q, 79a
thyroid, latent aberrant 78a
thyroid cancer 49q, 74a
    see also follicular thyroid carcinoma; medullary thyroid
        carcinoma; papillary thyroid carcinoma
thyroidectomy
    complications 54q, 77a
    counselling 59q, 79a
    permanent hypocalcaemia after 65q, 82a
    prophylactic 64q, 81–82a, 105a
thyroid eye disease, orbital decompression 56q, 78a

thyroid gland
  fine needle aspiration *see* fine needle aspiration (FNA) of thyroid
  swelling 53*q*, 76*a*
thyroid hormone synthesis 12*q*, 22*a*
thyroiditis 171*q*, 179*a*
  chronic lymphocytic 171*q*, 179*a*
  subacute granulomatous 171*q*, 179*a*
  subacute lymphocytic 171*q*, 179*a*
thyroid nodule
  possible follicular neoplasm 56*q*, 77*a*
  Thy 2 49*q*, 74*a*
  Thy 3 53*q*, 76*a*
  ultrasound features 66*q*, 83*a*
thyroplasty, injection 67*q*, 83*a*
tinnitus
  aspirin overdose 29*q*, 40*a*
  pulsatile 29*q*, 34*q*, 41*a*, 43*a*, 161*q*, 168*a*
TNM classification
  depth of tumour invasion 86*a*
  HPV/EBV-negative tumours 72*q*, 86*a*
  HPV-positive tonsillar carcinoma 84*a*
  lymph node metastases with unknown primary 72*q*, 86*a*
  maxillary sinus squamous cell carcinoma 109*q*, 126*a*
  nasopharyngeal carcinoma neck metastases 57*q*, 78*a*
  oral cavity tumours 71*q*, 86*a*
  pyriform fossa tumour 59*q*, 79*a*
  sinonasal malignancies 199*q*, 206*a*
  tonsillar carcinoma nodal metastases 48*q*, 73*a*
  tonsil tumours 72*q*, 86*a*
  see also American Joint Committee on Cancer (AJCC) staging
tongue carcinoma
  T1, management 71*q*, 85–86*a*
  TNM staging 71*q*, 86*a*
tonsillar carcinoma
  staging of HPV-positive 69*q*, 84*a*
  staging of lymph node metastases 48*q*, 73*a*
  TNM staging 72*q*, 86*a*
tonsillectomy
  parental consent 88*q*, 100*a*
  postoperative haemorrhage 89*q*, 90*q*, 101*a*
tonsillitis 189*q*, 194*a*
tonsils
  blood supply 14*q*, 23*a*, 66*q*, 82*a*
  enlarged, with persistent drooling 98*q*, 105*a*
toxoplasmosis, congenital 186*q*, 193*a*
tracheal stenosis
  airflow resistance 90*q*, 101*a*
  Myer–Cotton grading 91*q*, 102*a*
tracheo-oesophageal fistula 92*q*, 102*a*
tracheostomy
  national safety project 99*q*, 106*a*
  paediatric 97*q*, 105*a*
Trautman's triangle 34*q*, 43*a*

Treacher Collins syndrome 102*a*, 167*a*, 188*q*, 194*a*
Treponema pallidum 5*q*, 18*a*
Tri-adcortyl otic 162*q*, 168*a*
trigeminal nerve, ammonia sensitivity 110*q*, 126*a*
Trousseau sign 7*q*, 19*a*
Tumarkin crisis 158*q*, 165*a*
tympanic membrane, development 34*q*, 43*a*, 104*a*
tympanometry 159*q*, 166*a*
type I error 19*a*

U

ulcerative colitis 84*a*
ultrasound
  cervical lymphadenopathy 96*q*, 104*a*
  thyroid nodule 66*q*, 83*a*
upper aerodigestive tract
  development 91*q*, 102*a*
  granulomatous disorders 131–32*a*
upper respiratory tract infections, children 94*q*, 104*a*
urinary catheter, French scale 109*q*, 126*a*
Usher syndrome 91*q*, 102*a*
  clinical scenarios 158*q*, 165*a*
  hearing loss type 44*a*
  inheritance 190*q*, 195*a*
utricle 38*a*
uveoparotid disease (Heerfordt syndrome) 201*q*, 207*a*
uvulopalatopharyngoplasty (UVPP) 52*q*, 76*a*

V

vaccination, human papillomavirus 89*q*
vagal paraganglioma 37*q*, 45*a*
vagus nerve 16*a*
van der Woude syndrome 190*q*, 195*a*
vascular malformations, cutaneous capillary 92*q*, 102*a*
vertigo
  benign paroxysmal positional *see* benign paroxysmal positional vertigo
  hearing loss with 158*q*, 165*a*
  SCUBA diver 32*q*, 42*a*
vestibular evoked myogenic potentials (VEMPs)
  cervical (cVEMPs) 35*q*, 44*a*
  vestibulocollic reflex 26*q*, 38*a*
vestibular schwannoma *see* acoustic neuroma
vestibular system, anatomy 26*q*, 38*a*
vidian nerve 174*q*, 181*a*
vidian neurectomy 74*a*
visual reinforcement audiometry 33*q*, 43*a*, 166*a*, 192*a*
vitamin K 21*a*
vocal cords
  abductors 10*q*, 21*a*
  acute haemorrhage 48*q*, 73*a*
  drainage of oedema 54*q*
  layers 56*q*, 77*a*
  squamous cell carcinoma *see* laryngeal carcinoma
voice, fundamental frequency 76*a*

voice changes
    after drainage of vocal cord oedema 54q, 76a
    opera singer with 48q, 73a
    smoker with 53q, 76a
    spasmodic dysphonia 66q, 82a
    see also hoarseness
voice clinic, multidisciplinary team 54q, 77a
vomeronasal organ 17a
von Willebrand factor 21a

W

Waardenburg syndrome
    dystopia canthorum 36q, 44a, 102a
    inheritance 190q, 195a
    neonatal screening 190q, 195a
    type 2 158q, 165a
    type 4 158q, 165a
warfarin
    indications for reversal 10q, 21a
    mechanism of action 9q, 21a
Weerda technique 167a
Wegener granulomatosis see granulomatosis with
    polyangiitis

weight calculation, child 187q, 193a
Western blotting 145q, 152a
WETFLAG acronym 187q, 193a
windsurfer 36q, 45a
wood dust exposure 127a, 199q, 202q, 206a, 208a
World Health Organization (WHO), performance status
    (PS) 83–84a
wound healing
    facial skin 114q, 128a
    fibroblasts 115q, 128a

X

xeroderma pigmentosum 127a
X-rays
    child with history of choking 93q, 103a
    chronic throat discomfort 58q, 78a
    foreign body sensation on swallowing 60q, 79a
    hyperinflated lung 150a
Xylocaine, dental 147q, 154a

Z

Zitelli (bilobed) flap, dorsum of nose 117q, 129a
Z-plasty 114q, 128a

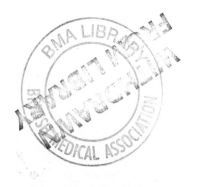